Survey of

Infectious
and
Parasitic Diseases

Kent M. Van De Graaff

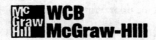
WCB
McGraw-Hill

Boston, Massachusetts   Burr Ridge, Illinois   Dubuque, Iowa
Madison, Wisconsin   New York, New York   San Francisco, California   St. Louis, Missouri

WCB/McGraw-Hill
A Division of The McGraw·Hill Companies

ISBN 0-697-27535-3

Printed in the United States of America

10 9

CONTENTS

Francis Bacon once said "A healthy body is a quest-chamber for the soul; a sick body is a prison." Because so many of the diseases that afflict humans are caused by microorganisms, it is important to learn about them. Infectious diseases can readily disrupt body homeostasis and result in sickness and frequently death. It is estimated by the World Health Organization (WHO), that tropical diseases kill more than 2 million people a year. These diseases are posing significant dangers to travelers. It is thought that deaths from tropical diseases will double over the next 20 years.

Infectious diseases are caused by microscopic organisms, such as certain viruses, protozoa, fungi, and bacteria. Parasitic diseases are transmitted by specific parasites, such as trematodes, cestodes, and nematodes. A mode of transmission is required in the spread of infectious diseases. In some diseases, there are specific vector organisms. These may be particular insects and other arthropods or specific parasites that transmit infectious microorganisms. Other infectious diseases are transmitted through the air, water, food, blood, or by direct contact.

A Survey of Infectious and Parasitic Diseases is intended to present the essential information about 100 of the most common and clinical significant diseases. Some of them (such as acne or the common cold) are not life-threatening but are never-the-less of clinical concern. Others are of immense importance because of the amount of suffering and death they cause each year. Cures are not available for many of these diseases. A page presentation is devoted to each of these diseases that includes a pronunciation, derivation, definition, life cycle, description, signs and symptoms, laboratory diagnosis, and prevention and treatment. Great care and preparation have gone into researching the life cycles of these diseases. These depictions are all new (not previously published) and informative. Chris H. Creek is the talented artist who rendered the life cycles and modes of infections for each of these diseases. I am most appreciative of his talent and his dedication to this project.

Acne (ack'nee) Gk. *acme*, point of efflorescence

DEFINITION: An inflammatory condition of the skin caused by the blockage and infection of sebaceous glands; occurs most frequently during puberty and adolescence. Individual lesions are commonly called pimples, whiteheads, or blackheads.

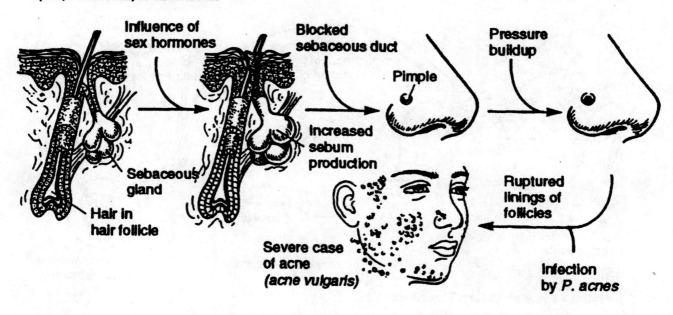

DESCRIPTION: More than 65% of adolescents any many adults suffer acne to some degree, making it the most common of the human skin diseases. Acne is a result of pubescent hormonal changes, especially increased levels of sex hormones (testosterone and, to a lesser extent, estrogen). Acne may also result from abnormal keratinization and obstruction in the sebaceous duct. Sex hormones stimulate sebum secretion from the sebaceous (oil) skin glands. The blockage of sebaceous ducts and the retention of sebum within the sebaceous glands causes the formation of first whiteheads then blackheads. Individual lesions usually occur on the face, upper back, and chest. If enough pressure builds up, the hair follicle lining may become ruptured allowing infection to occur. *Propionibacterium acnes*, a gram-positive, anaerobic, diphtheroid bacterium, commonly found in the skin, then breaks down the trapped sebum into free fatty acids. These acids can in turn trigger an inflammatory response of papules, pustules, and cysts leading to the more severe symptoms and possible scarring of *acne vulgaris*.

PREVENTION AND TREATMENT: Contrary to popular belief, diet does not have an appreciable effect on acne. Proper skin hygiene (including decreased use of makeup) and topical application of benzoyl peroxide are the most common methods of acne prevention. In extreme cases, tetracycline or accutane (a synthetic form of vitamin A) may be prescribed. "Picking" pimples is not a wise practice as it traumatizes the infection site, frequently rupturing the pimple inward and expanding the infection. It also increases the chances of scarring.

African Trypanosomiasis   Gk. *trypanon*, a borer; *soma*, body; *iasis*, infection

DEFINITION: An acute infectious disease characterized by marked lethargy, drowsiness, muscular weakness and cerebral symptoms; caused by a protozoan introduced into the blood by the bite of a tse-tse fly; also called *African sleeping sickness.*

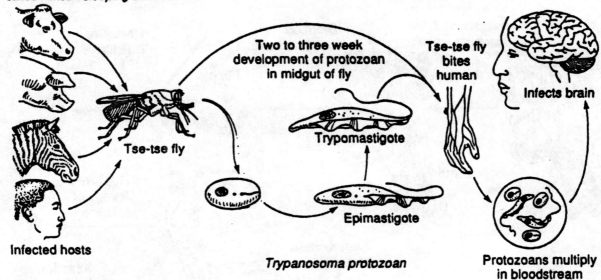

Infectious cycle of African Trypanosomiasis

DESCRIPTION: Described as a disease during the 14th century, African trypanosomiasis afflicts thousands of people yearly in Africa. In some villages 30–50% of the inhabitants are infected. *Rhodesian sleeping sickness* is endemic to east and central Africa and is caused by the protozoa *Trypanosoma brucei rhodesiense*. *Gambian sleeping sickness* is endemic to west and central Africa and is caused by *Trypanosoma brucei gambiense.* The pathogens for both kinds of trypanosomiasis are spindle-shaped protozoa which live in the blood plasma of the host. The bloodsucking tse-tse fly (*Glossina palpalis*) carrier becomes infected by ingesting the blood of a person or animal with the disease. The protozoan undergoes a two to three week cycle of development in the fly's midgut and then invades its salivary glands. The protozoa can be transferred as the infected fly bites its victim. Cattle, swine, and wild game animals may harbor the protozoa and are the reservoir of infection.

SIGNS AND SYMPTOMS: Initial symptoms of trypanosomiasis are fever, inflammation of the lymph nodes, and neck swelling. As the organisms multiply in the bloodstream and invade the brain of the victim, the symptoms include increased lethargy, weakness, muscle tremors, and anemia. An untreated victim will generally die from myocarditis or a secondary infection, such as pneumonia, within a year of contracting the disease.

LABORATORY DIAGNOSIS: Diagnosis is based on the microscopic observation of trypanosomes in the blood, cerebrospinal fluid, bone marrow or lymph node aspiration. CNS disease is manifested by pleocytosis and elevation of cerebrospinal fluid total protein and IgM levels.

PREVENTION AND TREATMENT: The most effective prevention is to avoid areas densely populated by the tse-tse fly vector or to spray and try to control the population of flies. Stream sides and waterholes are common areas inhabited by the tse-tse fly. It is also important to improve housing conditions in order to make them safer and more free of flies. There is no vaccination available for trypanosomiasis and protective immunity does not develop with an infection. Treatment during the hemolymphatic stage of the disease includes the administering of the drugs suramin or pentamidine isethionate. Melarsoprol is recommended in patients who have progressed to the stage of neurological affliction.

AIDS (Acquired Immunodeficiency Syndrome)

DEFINITION: A disease of the immune system in which T-helper (T_H) cell numbers are greatly reduced due to infection by human immunodeficiency virus (HIV). Death from AIDS is often due to secondary infection by other opportunistic microorganisms.

Transmission of HIV

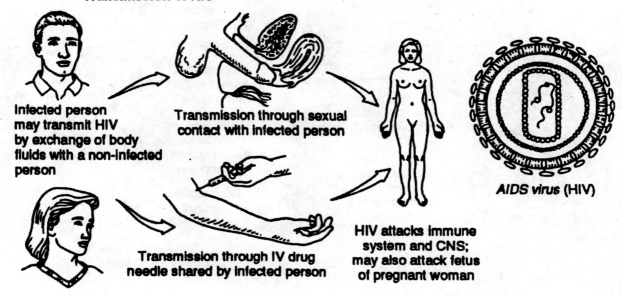

Infected person may transmit HIV by exchange of body fluids with a non-infected person

Transmission through sexual contact with infected person

Transmission through IV drug needle shared by infected person

HIV attacks immune system and CNS; may also attack fetus of pregnant woman

AIDS virus (HIV)

DESCRIPTION: AIDS is one possible result of infection by the human immunodeficiency virus, HIV. HIV is a *retrovirus* which is transmitted in body fluids. HIV attacks T_4(CD_4) cells (including T_H cells, necessary in the immune response); stopping their cell division, and occasionally killing them. Because HIV also invades monocytes and macrophage cells, it is able to infect the central nervous system (CNS) of an AIDS victim and the fetus of a pregnant woman with AIDS. With T_H cells repressed, the body becomes susceptible to other diseases. AIDS was first diagnosed in the U.S. in 1981 and has spread rapidly; there are currently over 2 million HIV carriers in the U.S. The rate is as high as 20% in some African countries. Most carriers are unaware they have the disease since the time between infection and AIDS symptoms can be long—up to 7 years or longer. HIV has a high frequency of antigenic drift, allowing it to change at a rapid pace.

SIGNS AND SYMPTOMS: Within 6 months after infection, the patient undergoes seroconversion. Symptoms at this early stage of infection include a mild fever, enlarged lymph nodes, and fatigue. These symptoms spontaneously disappear in a few weeks. Later, lymphadenopathy reappears, lasting for, perhaps, several years. The T_4 cells steadily decline in numbers to levels below 400 per ml. Immune responsiveness declines. Weight loss is common. AIDS is characterized by frequent and severe infections of *Candida albicans*, *Pneumocystis* pneumonia, various viruses, toxoplasmosis, and many others. Kaposi's sarcoma is common. CNS involvement may lead to dementia.

LABORATORY DIAGNOSIS: The initial step involves detection of IgG anti-HIV antibody in the patient's serum using an ELISA test. Positive antibody tests are confirmed by Western blotting.

PREVENTION AND TREATMENT: Since AIDS is sexually transmitted, abstinence or fidelity are the best ways to avoid contraction of the disease. In the absence of these conditions, avoidance of anal sex, sex without condoms, and sex with high-risk people (homosexuals, prostitutes, and IV drug users) is necessary. Since AIDS is also transmitted in blood, use of non-sterile or used needles should be avoided. Units of blood are screened for HIV antibody before being used for transfusion. HIV cannot be transmitted through casual contact. Since illness and death are caused by secondary disease, treatment of AIDS patients mostly consists of keeping other diseases under control. The current drug of choice for treating HIV itself is azidothymidine (AZT). AZT inhibits reverse transcriptase, an enzyme necessary for HIV replication. Although AZT appears to slow down AIDS, it does not cure the disease. Recently, AZT-resistant strains of HIV have been discovered.

DEFINITION: An inflammation of the colon caused by ingesting contaminated food or water containing the cysts of the amoeba *Entamoeba histolytica*; also known as *amoebiasis*.

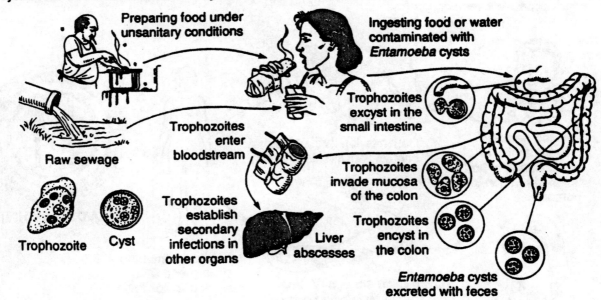

DESCRIPTION: Amebic dysentery is contracted by eating food or drinking water contaminated with cysts from the protozoan *Entamoeba histolytica*. Once ingested, trophozoites excyst (release) in the small intestine and then pass into the large intestine where they ulcerate the mucosa. In serious and prolonged cases of the disease, the trophozoites may enter the bloodstream and establish secondary infection sites (abscesses) such as in the liver or brain. Amebic dysentery is a world-health problem especially in countries that have poor sanitation and inadequate hygiene. An estimated 10% of the world population are carriers of the cysts, and 1% of these die from the disease. Trophozoites of *E. histolytica* reproduce by binary fission. The cysts are approximately 10 μm in diameter and possess four nuclei.

SIGNS AND SYMPTOMS: Nausea, intestinal dysentery, and colitis are the most common symptoms of amebic dysentery. Intestinal ulceration will soon develop in untreated persons, causing mucus and blood to appear in the feces.

LABORATORY DIAGNOSIS: Because *E. histolytica* is the only parasitic amoeba to engulf erythrocytes, their presence within examined trophozoites from stool dysenteric (not diarrheic) samples provides evidence for identification of the disease. Serological tests, including latex agglutination and fluorescent antibody tests, are used.

PREVENTION AND TREATMENT: Appropriate sanitation and personal hygiene are effective deterrents of the disease. Tourists to third-world countries should take precautions to avoid consuming contaminated food and water. Properly cooked foods are generally safe because amebic cysts are killed by cooking. Processed beverages are usually safe. Metronidazole plus iodoquinol are the drugs generally used in the treatment of amebic dysentery.

American Trypanosomiasis (Chagas' Disease) from Carlos Chagas, Brazilian physician, 1879–1934

DEFINITION: Disease caused by the protozoan *Trypanosoma cruzi* and transmitted to humans by the reduviid, or "kissing bug." Cases are mainly confined to poorer, rural areas of Latin America, particularly Brazil.

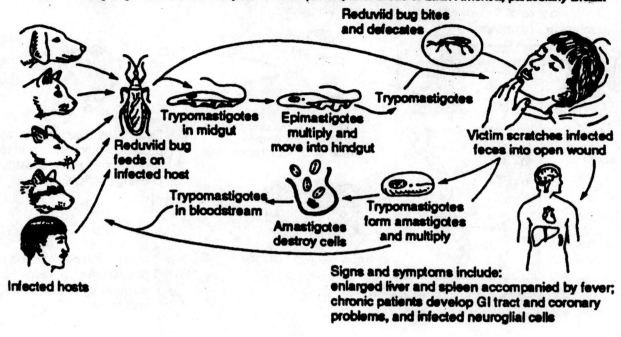

DESCRIPTION: A reduviid bug becomes infected by feeding on the blood of an infected human or other animal. During the next 2 weeks, the ingested *T. cruzi* trypomastigote multiplies in the insect's gut. Reduviid bugs live in the walls of mud structures and feed at night, typically by dropping from the ceiling and biting a sleeping person. They are called "kissing bugs" because they generally bite about the lips or eyelids. As a bug feeds, it defecates, and the trypomastigote is shed in the feces. When the human awakens and scratches the area of the bite, he introduces infectious feces into the open wound. A lesion known as a *chagoma* is formed at the site, and the trypomastigotes spread throughout the body via the bloodstream, concentrating in myocardial, glial, and reticuloendothelial cells. Within these host cells, the organisms form nonflagellated amastigotes which multiply and eventually destroy the cell to re-enter the bloodstream. There they differentiate into trypomastigotes which may be taken up by the reduviid bug, completing the cycle. Dogs, cats, rats, and raccoons may also serve as the reservoir for *T. cruzi*, and the reduviid bug is also the vector for their infection.

SIGNS AND SYMPTOMS: Acute infection is manifested by fever, and enlargement of the liver and spleen resolving within 2 months, but is often asymptomatic. A few patients develop chronic disease, manifested by an inflammatory reaction in the heart, where signs may include myocarditis, heart enlargement, or heart failure, or in the GI tract, manifested as megaesophagus or megacolon.

LABORATORY DIAGNOSIS: Acute disease is diagnosed by demonstrating trypomastigotes in smears of the patient's blood, but this is often difficult because the organisms are never very numerous. Xenodiagnosis is an effective means of diagnosis in which non-infected reduviid bugs are allowed to feed on the patient, and are later examined for presence of *T. cruzi* in the intestinal contents. Serology may also be helpful.

PREVENTION AND TREATMENT: Prevention involves controlling insects and improving housing conditions. No vaccine is available. Treatment with nifurtimox is only partially effective in the acute stage of the disease since it kills trypomastigotes in the blood, but is not effective against amastigotes in body tissues. Because there is no good remedy for either stage of the disease, a patient is treated symptomatically.

Anthrax (an'thraks) Gk. *anthrax,* charcoal

DEFINITION: An acute, infectious disease of ungulates (hoofed mammals). Humans may contract it through contact with infected animal hair, hides, or wastes. Death may result from depression of the respiratory centers due to toxin of *Bacillus anthracis,* the causative organism.

Transmission of anthrax

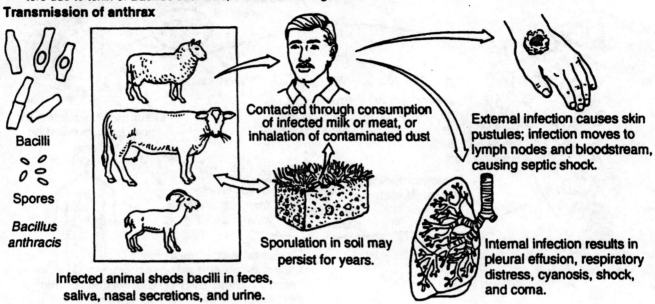

Bacilli

Spores

Bacillus anthracis

Infected animal sheds bacilli in feces, saliva, nasal secretions, and urine.

Contacted through consumption of infected milk or meat, or inhalation of contaminated dust

Sporulation in soil may persist for years.

External infection causes skin pustules; infection moves to lymph nodes and bloodstream, causing septic shock.

Internal infection results in pleural effusion, respiratory distress, cyanosis, shock, and coma.

DESCRIPTION: *Bacillus anthracis* is a gram-positive, spore-forming rod. Domestic animals are infected with anthrax through the intestine after grazing in spore-contaminated pastures. The bacillus regenerates and reproduces in the bloodstream. It can then be transmitted through infected milk or under-cooked meat. Humans can also contract the disease by inhaling dust containing spores or by direct contact through a cut or abrasion. Persons with occupations handling wools, hides, and animal brushes are at risk for infection. Large numbers of bacilli produce a sufficient amount of toxin to depress the respiratory centers within the brainstem, which is the usual cause of death.

SIGNS AND SYMPTOMS: With an external infection, a pustule or boil forms on the skin that is characterized by a red, edematous area surrounding a central blackened pit. Internal infections usually spread through the blood to regional lymph nodes. Untreated patients may experience septicemia, pleural effusion, respiratory distress, cyanosis, and eventually shock and coma.

LABORATORY DIAGNOSIS: Diagnostic techniques include culture of *B. anthracis* from vesicular fluids, exudates, or blood. Serological diagnosis by the ELISA test demonstrates a significant antibody titer.

PREVENTION AND TREATMENT: Prophylactic vaccination of livestock against anthrax is available. A vaccine containing attenuated bacteria is quite successful in cattle and sheep. An anthrax vaccine also exists for workers exposed to the disease. Animals that have been infected must be separated from the herd and the pasture disinfected by burning. Milk or meat from infected animals must be properly discarded. Animals that die from the disease should be completely cremated. The dressings of external lesions must also be burned. Animal hides, hair, and wool can be decontaminated by formaldehyde, gamma irradiation, steam under pressure, or ethylene oxide. Drug therapy includes erythromycin, tetracycline, or chloramphenicol.

Argentine Hemorrhagic Fever (AHF)

DEFINITION: A hemorrhagic fever which infects mainly farm workers in northwestern Argentina; caused by a rodent-borne *arenavirus* commonly called the *Junin virus*.

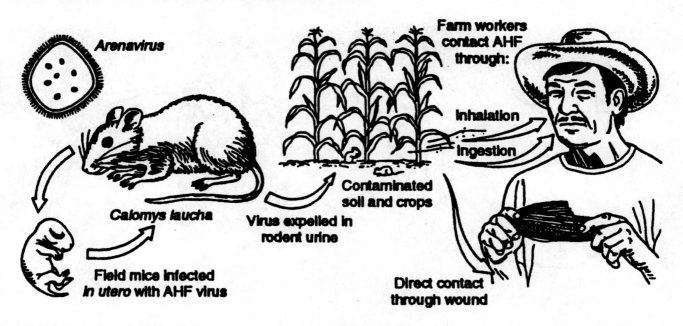

Arenavirus

Farm workers contact AHF through:

Inhalation

Ingestion

Calomys laucha

Contaminated soil and crops

Virus expelled in rodent urine

Field mice infected *in utero* with AHF virus

Direct contact through wound

DESCRIPTION: The single-stranded RNA virus which causes Argentine hemorrhagic fever (AHF) is spherical or pleomorphic, and 110–130 nm in diameter. Field mice, specifically *Calomys musculinus* and *Calomys laucha* are the natural reservoirs for this virus. These rodents acquire a chronic infection with AHF *in utero* and shed virus particles in the saliva and urine throughout life. Humans may contract the virus through cuts in the skin when handling crops contaminated by infected rodent urine, by eating contaminated food, or by inhaling contaminated dust. For this reason, the virus predominantly affects adult men working in the fields during the corn harvest. Human to human transmission of the virus is rare. AHF exhibits an incubation period of 6 to 14 days and the lymphatic tissues are the primary sites of viral replication. Other body tissues may be infected, including those of the heart, liver, and kidneys.

SIGNS AND SYMPTOMS: High fever, retro-orbital pain, nausea, vomiting, and a rash on the upper body are noted in the first 3 to 4 days of the illness. Between days 4 and 6, hemorrhage appears in the form of inflamed conjunctivae, nosebleeds, and bleeding gums. Approximately 75% of AHF patients improve rapidly after day 7 and recover without permanent problems during 1 to 3 months convalescence. After day 7, severe cases involving the central nervous system are characterized by confusion, irritability, and tremors of the hands and tongue. Death follows progression to delirium, convulsions, and coma in 10 to 15% of these cases.

LABORATORY DIAGNOSIS: Junin virus can be isolated in vero cells from blood, cerebrospinal fluid, and throat washings. Serological diagnosis is made by the immunofluorescence test. Detection of IgM is useful for early and rapid diagnosis.

PREVENTION AND TREATMENT: Although some progress has been made toward a vaccine, no effective method currently exists for preventing AHF. Rodent control is impractical because the virus hosts are so widely distributed in rural Argentina. Transfusion with immune plasma within 8 days after the onset of symptoms is the most effective treatment, reducing mortality to less than 2%.

Blastomycosis Gk. *blasto*, germ; *mykes*, fungus

DEFINITION: A disease that starts as a respiratory infection and spreads to the skin, bones, and other organs. There are North American, South American, and European strains of blastomycosis.

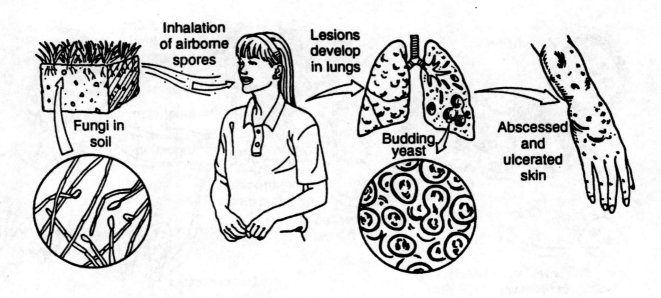

DESCRIPTION: Blastomycosis is the designation of three separate respiratory infections: *North American blastomycosis*, caused by the fungus *Blastomyces dermatitidis*; *South American blastomycosis*, caused by the fungus *Paracoccidiodes brasiliensis*; and *European blastomycosis*, caused by *Cryptococcus neoformans*. Of the three types, the South American blastomycosis is the most serious. South American blastomycosis is a chronic, fatal mycosis with ulcerative granulomas of the buccal and nasal mucosa. Ulcerations occur in the lungs and on the skin, followed by lymphatic tissue inflammation and tissue destruction in other organs including the spleen and liver.

North American blastomycosis is generally not severe and accounts for between 30 and 60 deaths per year. The causative agent, *Blastomyces dermatitidis* is a dimorphic fungus—in soil it grows as a filamentous mold, while in an infected human it grows as a budding yeast. Spores from the fungus enter the body through the respiratory tract infecting the lungs and causing lesions similar to those of tuberculosis. From there it frequently spreads to the skin, forming abscesses and ulcerations. It may also invade the lymphatic, skeletal, reproductive, and urinary systems.

LABORATORY DIAGNOSIS: Diagnosis can be made by direct microscopic examination of biologic specimens digested in 10% KOH. Characteristic single-budding yeasts may be seen.

PREVENTION AND TREATMENT: Because fungal spores are spread through the wind and gain access to the respiratory tract through inhalation, it is advisable to avoid being out-of-doors on dusty, windy days. Like most other systemic fungi infections, blastomycosis is generally treated with Amphotericin B. Because Amphotericin B is a toxic agent, it often induces nausea, pain, and headaches as possible side effects to the patient.

Botulism (bot′u′lizm) L. *botulus*, sausage; Gk. *ismos*, condition

DEFINITION: A severe form of poisoning primarily from food containing one of the botulinal toxins produced by *Clostridium botulinum*, which is a gram-positive, anaerobic, spore-forming rod.

Some features of botulinal exotoxins

Toxin	Geographic location	Relative toxicity	Mortality rate
Type A	Western U.S.	4+	60–70%
Type B	Europe, Eastern U.S.	3+	25%
Type E	Pacific, Northwest, Alaska, Great Lakes	3+	40%

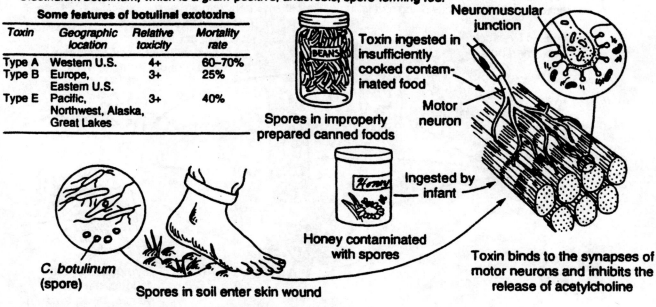

Spores in improperly prepared canned foods

Toxin ingested in insufficiently cooked contaminated food

Honey contaminated with spores

Ingested by infant

C. botulinum (spore)

Spores in soil enter skin wound

Neuromuscular junction

Motor neuron

Toxin binds to the synapses of motor neurons and inhibits the release of acetylcholine

Modes of transmission of *Clostridium botulinum*

DESCRIPTION: The neurotoxin produced by *Clostridium botulinum* is one of the most poisonous substances known, and even minute quantities can be lethal. The spores of *Clostridium botulinum* are commonly found in the soil and contaminate improperly processed food. An anaerobic environment stimulates the spores to germinate, and the multiplying bacilli produce the botulinal toxin. Once ingested, the toxin affects neuromuscular junctions by inhibiting the release of acetylcholine in muscle stimulation.

SIGNS AND SYMPTOMS: The initial symptoms are ptosis of the facial muscles, blurred or double vision, dysphagia (difficulty swallowing), and a dry sore throat. Untreated victims experience weakness and fatigue, followed by flaccid paralysis which may lead to quadriplegia and respiratory failure. Death is usually due to asphyxia.

LABORATORY DIAGNOSIS: Mice are inoculated with patient samples (serum, vomitus, stool) or food samples. Immune mice are protected while non-immunized animals die, showing the toxin to be botulinal toxin. Typing of the toxin is also done in this manner.

PREVENTION AND TREATMENT: The toxin can be denatured by heating food at 80° C (or 201° F) for ten minutes. Canned and preserved foods such as vegetables and meats (e.g., sausages) should be considered as possible botulism vehicles, so proper cooking before consumption is advisable. Original processing at 120° C (273° F) will inactivate all spores. Babies under one year old should not be given honey because the *C. botulinum* spores in contaminated honey can readily multiply in a baby's GI tract, causing infant botulism.

Treatment of botulism poisoning requires the removal of stomach contents to eliminate residual toxin. This is followed by the administration of an antitoxin, but hypersensitivity to horse proteins must first be assessed. In seriously ill patients, artificial respiration or a tracheostomy may be needed. Although recovery is slow, it is usually complete if the patient has proper medical treatment.

Brucellosis from Sir David Bruce, Scottish microbiologist, 1855–1931

DEFINITION: An infectious bacterial disease characterized by fever, sweating, weakness, and joint aches. Caused by *Brucella* species, it may be chronic and produce long-lasting disability; also known as *undulant fever*, because of the repetitious rising and falling of the patient's body temperature.

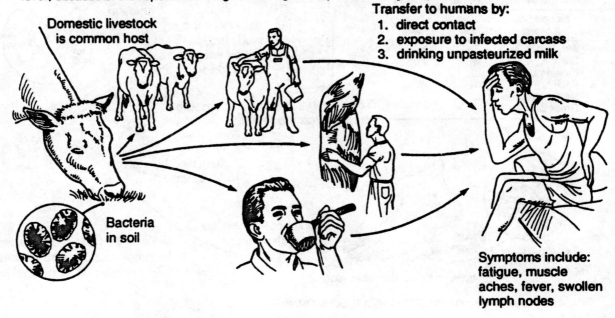

Domestic livestock is common host

Bacteria in soil

Transfer to humans by:
1. direct contact
2. exposure to infected carcass
3. drinking unpasteurized milk

Symptoms include: fatigue, muscle aches, fever, swollen lymph nodes

DESCRIPTION: *Brucella* is a genus of bacteria characterized as small (1μm), gram-negative, aerobic rods. There are five principal species: *B. melitensis, abortus, suis, canis,* and *ovis*—infecting goats, cattle, swine, dogs, and sheep respectively, *Brucella abortus* grows actively on the placenta of a pregnant cow causing an abortion of its fetus but not the placenta. The infected cow becomes unable to bear additonal young because of the retention of the attached diseased placenta on the uterine wall. Although normally transmitted from animal to animal, all of these species are also infectious to humans. Brucellosis is particularly hazardous to farmers, veterinarians, and slaughter-house workers. The organism may be spread from animal to humans in infected dairy products, direct contact with diseased animals, or exposure to their carcasses. Once in the body, the organisms survive ingestion by macrophages (thereby gaining protection from the immune system) and may spread throughout the lymphatic and circulatory system.

SIGNS AND SYMPTOMS: The symptoms of brucellosis in humans include weakness, general malaise, backache, headache, loss of appetite, swollen lymph nodes, and undulating fever. In more serious cases, nodes form in bone marrow, the endocardium, and along the meninges of the brain. Approximately 200 cases of brucellosis are diagnosed in the U.S. each year, and the mortality rate is relatively low.

LABORATORY DIAGNOSIS: Diagnosis is based on serology. An agglutination test is used to detect antibodies in animals and humans. ELISA testing is also used, which is more sensitive and specific. Infected individuals show as antibody-positive.

PREVENTION AND TREATMENT: The most effective preventions are slaughtering affected animals (identified by serotesting) and burning their carcasses, immunizing young animals, and pasteurizing milk and milk products. Persons afflicted with Brucellosis have a mortality rate of 3% if untreated, and full recovery if treated. Untreated survivors, however, generally have chronic symptoms. Treatment consists of tetracycline and streptomycin therapy for 3 to 4 weeks.

Candidiasis (can-did-i'ah-sis) L. *candidus*, dazzling white

DEFINITION: An infection with or disease caused by the yeast, *Candida albicans*. This includes oral (thrush), vulvovaginal, cutaneous, gastrointestinal, and systemic candidiasis.

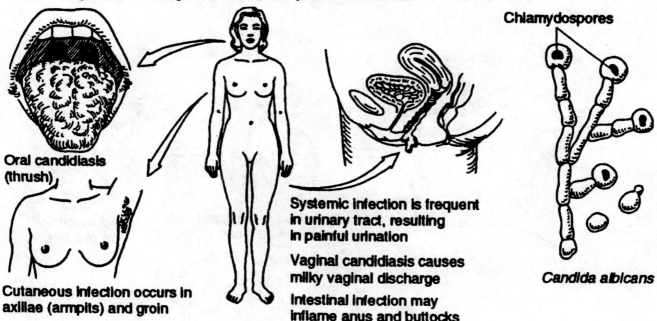

Oral candidiasis (thrush)

Cutaneous infection occurs in axillae (armpits) and groin

Systemic infection is frequent in urinary tract, resulting in painful urination

Vaginal candidiasis causes milky vaginal discharge

Intestinal infection may inflame anus and buttocks

Chlamydospores

Candida albicans

DESCRIPTION: *Candida albicans* is a common fungus in the environment, including the surface of the skin, body orifices (openings), and GI tract. It is a part of the naturally occurring microbial population. It is primarily when body immunity is weakened, body fluids are abnormally changed (increased sugar content in urine, altered pH or hormonal levels), or when the normal body flora are altered that the organism multiplies and candidiasis develops. The cultured yeast has numerous filaments called *pseudohyphae*. Candidiasis of the oropharynx, vulva, vagina, and GI tract is common, and the symptoms depend upon the location of the infection.

SIGNS AND SYMPTOMS: *Oral candidiasis*, commonly called *thrush*, exhibits a creamy gray membrane covering the tongue. Newborns commonly contract it by exposure to *C. albicans* in the vagina during parturition. *Vaginal candidiasis* is one cause of *vulvovaginitis*, and is characterized by a curd-like, milky vaginal discharge. *Cutaneous candidiasis* usually occurs in the axillae (armpits), groin, or other moist body areas. *Gastrointestinal candidiasis* frequently causes swelling of the anus and buttocks. *Systemic candidiasis* may cause urinary tract infections, endocarditis, and meningitis.

LABORATORY DIAGNOSIS: Candidiasis is diagnosed by microscopic examination of exudates, scraping of lesions, and by isolation of the fungus in culture.

PREVENTION AND TREATMENT: Since *C. albicans* is an opportunistic organism, candidiasis generally results when the body's defenses and competing microorganisms' numbers are down. This could result from pregnancy, diabetes, antibiotic treatments, prolonged systemic diseases, AIDS, etc. Oral, vulvovaginal, and cutaneous candidiasis are normally treated with nystatin as an ointment or suppository. Candicidin is an alternative drug. Amphotericin B is generally used to treat systemic and gastrointestinal candidiasis.

Canine Parvovirus L. *canis*, dog

DEFINITION: A viral disease of dogs characterized by severe diarrhea and leukopenia. The causative agent is a parvovirus characterized by a single-stranded DNA genome, no envelope, icosahedral symmetry, and nuclear replication.

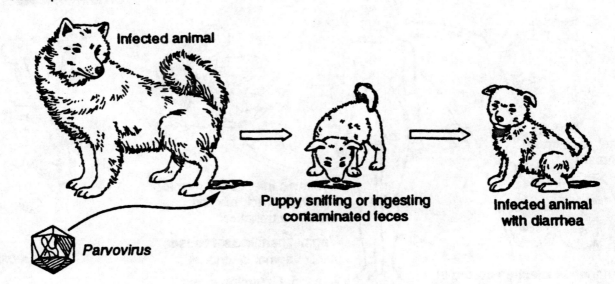

DESCRIPTION: Canine parvoviral infection afflicts dogs throughout the world. The virus itself is similar to feline panleukopenia (a viral cat disease). The disease is spread through ingested canine feces and contaminated kennels and soil. The parvovirus causing the disease may be viable for a year outside a dog's body.
   The parvovirus is extremely small (about 20 nm) has a single-stranded DNA genome, icosahedral symmetry, and no envelope. DNA replication and capsid formulation occur in the nuclei of host animal cells. The parvovirus is heat resistant, being able to survive temperatures of up to 60° C for half an hour.

SIGNS AND SYMPTOMS: The virus attacks mitotically active cells, especially those lining the GI tract and within red bone marrow. The principal symptoms of canine parvoviral infection are severe diarrhea, vomiting, myocarditis, and leukopenia (decreased leukocytes in the bloodstream). Because of damage to the lining of the small intestine, pups with canine parvovirus become severely dehydrated in one to two days and frequently die a few days later if untreated.

LABORATORY DIAGNOSIS: Diagnosis can be made serologically by detecting anti-viral antibodies using hemagglutination inhibition, immunofluorescence, or serum neutralization tests; also by virus isolation in canine or feline cell lines.

PREVENTION AND TREATMENT: Since pups are most affected by the parvovirus, vaccination between weaning and the age of 18 weeks is advised. Infected dogs are intravenously given nutrients and electrolytes to replace those lost by diarrhea. This treatment usually takes three to four days, and the survival rate is high for treated animals.

Cellulitis (sel-u-li'tis) L. *cella*, chamber; GK, *Itis*, inflammation

DEFINITION: An inflammatory infiltration of tissues that spreads along fasciae and in spaces between muscles. This diffuse, ill-defined spreading lesion is most commonly caused by Group A streptococci and *Staphylococcus aureus*.

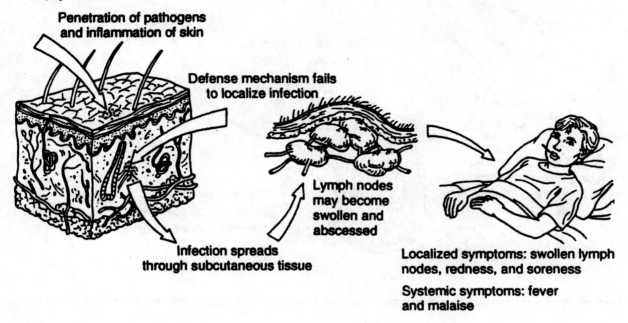

Penetration of pathogens and inflammation of skin

Defense mechanism fails to localize infection

Infection spreads through subcutaneous tissue

Lymph nodes may become swollen and abscessed

Localized symptoms: swollen lymph nodes, redness, and soreness

Systemic symptoms: fever and malaise

DESCRIPTION: Quick acting body defense mechanisms will usually localize an infection in the skin or close to the skin. If an inflammation spreads through the deep subcutaneous tissue, however, the condition is called *cellulitis*. This condition is more common in children than in adults. Hospitalization may become necessary if the inflammatory process is extensive enough to cause serious systemic effects. In addition to Group A streptococci and the staphylococci, *Haemophilis influenzae* may cause cellulitis. Necrotizing fasciitis (a form of cellulitis) is caused by a mixture of aerobic and anaerobic gram-negative organisms.

SIGNS AND SYMPTOMS: An inflammation of the skin and subcutaneous tissues occurs with intense redness, swelling, and firm infiltration. It is not uncommon for the regional lymph nodes to become swollen. The infection may progress to abscess formation. Depending on the extent of the spreading, systemic effects include varying degrees of fever and malaise. The orbital area of the face is a frequent site of cellulitis, thus creating the possibility that complications of paranasal sinusitis and meningitis could occur.

LABORATORY DIAGNOSIS: Diagnosis may be made by culture under aerobic and/or anaerobic conditions. Isolates are tested for antibiotic sensitivity.

PREVENTION AND TREATMENT: Oral or parenteral penicillin, erythromycin, dicloxacillin, or the cephalosporins are the usual drugs of choice. Patient rest and immobilization of the affected area are also recommended techniques to decrease inflammation and to inhibit spreading. Hot, moist compresses to the infected area can speed blood flow and also reduce inflammation. A method for prevention of the initial spread of inflammation is not known.

Chancroid (shan'kroyd) L. *cancer;* Gk. *eidos,* resemblance

DEFINITION: A sexually transmitted disease (STD) that causes genital ulcers and swollen regional lymph nodes; caused by the bacterium *Hemophilus ducreyi.*

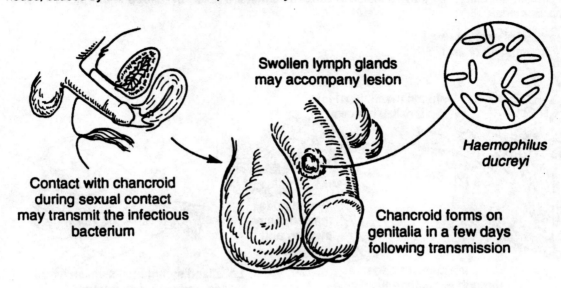

Swollen lymph glands may accompany lesion

Contact with chancroid during sexual contact may transmit the infectious bacterium

Chancroid forms on genitalia in a few days following transmission

Haemophilus ducreyi

DESCRIPTION: Chancroid is the result of genital infection by the gram-negative bacterium, *Hemophilus ducreyi.* Chancroid is sexually transmitted, with a time lapse of 3 to 7 days between infection and the appearance of symptoms. The disease occurs most commonly in tropical areas including Africa, the Caribbean, and Southeast Asia. In the United States, there are approximately 5,000 reported cases each year.

SIGNS AND SYMPTOMS: The principal sign is the appearance of painful chancroids (soft chancres, not unlike those of the first stage of syphilis). Often, lymph nodes in the area become swollen, and may eventually break through to the surface, discharging highly infectious pus. Individual lesions are able to infect the surrounding area, causing multiple lesions in many victims. Lesions may also occur on the tongue or lips having been contracted during oral sex. The appearance of the lesions may be confused with the lesions of primary syphilis or genital herpes, therefore, differential diagnosis may be required. If untreated, the lesions may persist for months and leave deep scarring.

LABORATORY DIAGNOSIS: Smears obtained from the lesions reveal small, gram-negative bacilli upon microscopic examination. Positive cultures can be obtained in over 80% of cases. The medium of choice is chocolate agar containing 3 µg/ml of vancomycin.

PREVENTION AND TREATMENT: The best method of prevention is to avoid sexual contact with infected people. Using condoms is only effective when used appropriately and when the condom is able to cover or protect from *all* lesions. A variety of antibacterial agents may be used to treat the disease, including erythromycin, tetracycline, or sulfa drugs.

Chicken Pox (Varicella) L. *varicella*, a tiny spot

DEFINITION: An acute, highly contagious viral disease occurring most frequently in children. It presents a typical blister-like rash which is more concentrated on the trunk of the body; caused by the *varicella-zoster virus,* a member of the herpes virus family.

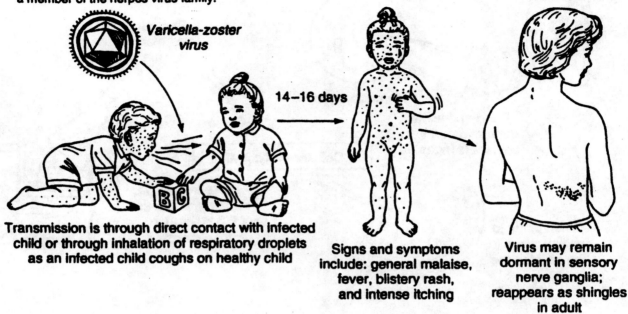

Varicella-zoster virus

14–16 days

Transmission is through direct contact with infected child or through inhalation of respiratory droplets as an infected child coughs on healthy child

Signs and symptoms include: general malaise, fever, blistery rash, and intense itching

Virus may remain dormant in sensory nerve ganglia; reappears as shingles in adult

DESCRIPTION: Humans are the only known host of chicken pox. Epidemics are most frequent in temperate zones during the winter and spring months. Varicella-zoster viruses are present in the fluid of most blisters and also in the respiratory tract. The disease is transmitted by inhalation or direct contact. The virus then multiplies in the respiratory epithelium and disseminates via the blood to the skin of the trunk and face. Chicken pox has a 14–16 day incubation period, so carriers may transmit the disease before they realize that they have it. Adults without immunity who contract the disease have more severe cases than children. Though a minor childhood disease, the virus may remain in a latent state in sensory nerve ganglia and later reappear in a reactivated form called *shingles.* Encephalitis is a rare but serious possible complication of both primary infection and shingles.

SIGNS AND SYMPTOMS: A blistery rash on the face and trunk, accompanied by fever, intense itching, and general malaise is common. Secondary bacterial infections may occur due to scratching of the rash areas. The vesicles and blisters crust over and heal with occasional scarring.

LABORATORY DIAGNOSIS: Diagnosis is made serologically by demonstrating IgM anti-viral antibody using ELISA tests. Antibody titers in paired sera may demonstrate current infection. Isolation of virus from lesion exudates and nasopharyngeal specimens in cell culture is diagnostic of primary and reactivation infection.

PREVENTION AND TREATMENT: Chicken pox usually stimulates a level of lifelong antibody response that prevents subsequent attacks. There is no generally administered vaccine. High risk immunocompromised infants and children with documented exposure may, however, be given temporary protection through injections of varicella-zoster immune globulin. Sick children should be kept from school and from contact with other susceptible children for one week or until six days after the last vesicle group appears. Chicken pox may be especially threatening to immunosuppressed patients or elderly individuals.

Cholera (kol'er-a) L. *cholera*, bilious diarrhea

DEFINITION: An acute infection of the small intestine, characterized by profuse, watery diarrhea and vomiting; caused by the bacterium *Vibrio cholerae*. Humans are the only known host.

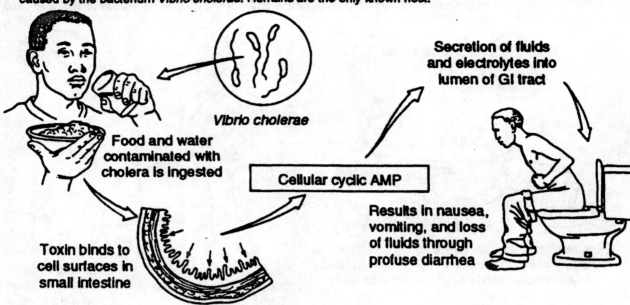

DESCRIPTION: The *Vibrio cholerae* bacteria are slightly curved, gram-negative rods with single polar flagella. They may be ingested in food or water that has been contaminated by infected feces. The bacteria attach to the mucosa in the small intestine where they release an enterotoxin called *choleragen*. The toxin binds to cell surfaces and activates the production of adenyl cyclase causing a great increase in cellular cyclic AMP that promotes the secretion of fluid and electrolytes into the lumen of the gut. The result is diarrhea and extreme loss of fluids and electrolytes from the body. Cholera is common in areas of poor sanitation with 100,000–200,000 cases reported throughout the world each year.

SIGNS AND SYMPTOMS: Early symptoms of cholera include nausea, vomiting, abdominal cramping, and profuse diarrhea. The watery diarrhea is referred to as a "rice-water stool." Because 10–20 liters of fluid a day may be lost, severe dehydration occurs rapidly resulting in an increased pulse and respiration and a low or absent blood pressure. Other symptoms of prolonged disease include sunken eyes and cheeks and wrinkled skin. Hypovolemic shock may develop usually resulting in death. A 70% mortality exists in untreated cases.

LABORATORY DIAGNOSIS: The cholera bacteria can be readily cultured from infected feces in alkaline media.

PREVENTION AND TREATMENT: Education, early detection, treatment of carriers, and sanitation (especially of the water) are the most important prevention techniques. Patient treatment consists of vigorous replacement of lost fluids and electrolytes (orally or intravenously). Infection with *V. cholerae* results in a short-lived immunity of only 4–12 months. Vaccination also provides short duration of protection. Tetracycline is used to kill bacteria and decrease toxin formation.

Coccidioidomycosis L. *coccoid*, sphere; *mycosis*, fungal infection

DEFINITION: A deep mycotic infection of the respiratory tract caused by the fungus, *Coccidioides immitis*; also known as *San Joaquin Valley Fever*

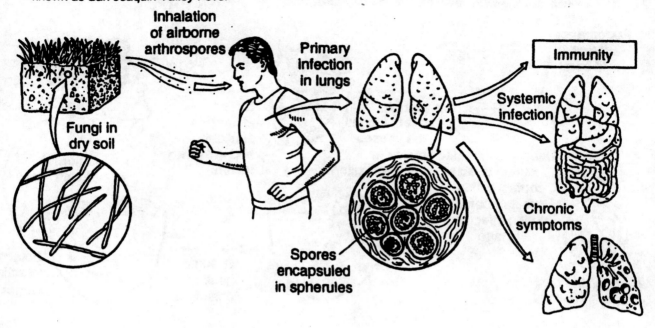

DESCRIPTION: *Coccidioides immitis* is a dimorphic fungus native to the southwest U.S., Mexico, and South America. The spores are found in dry and highly alkaline soil. When in the soil, the fungus exists in a septate mycelial form that produces arthrospores. The arthrospores are barrel-shaped structures about 20 μm to 60 μm in diameter, which may become airborne attached to dust particles. Inhaled arthrospores form thick-walled spherules within the bronchioles and alveoli of the lungs. Within a few weeks, cell-mediated immunity appears to the spherules. Some of the spherules may spread to other body organs and others may break down into several hundred spores. When the spores are released in the environment and settle in the soil, each can form a germ tube and then another septate mycelium.

It is estimated that 100,000 people each year contract coccidioidomycosis, with 50–100 fatalities. In the U.S., the disease is most common in the southwest deserts of California and Arizona. Once a person has been exposed to the fungus, resistance to further infection is established.

SIGNS AND SYMPTOMS: Most people who contract coccidioidomycosis are asymptomatic. In others, the symptoms include chest pain, fever, malaise, dry cough, and some weight loss. In more severe cases, the symptoms are indistinguishable from tuberculosis.

LABORATORY DIAGNOSIS: The organism is readily cultured from fluids or lesions and spherules can be found by direct examination of fluids or tissues. Skin testing, which detects delayed hypersensitivity, distinguishes between coccidioidomycosis and tuberculosis.

PREVENTION AND TREATMENT: It is advisable in the arid environment of southwestern U.S. to avoid being out-of-doors on windy days. Fortunately, for most people who contract coccidioidomycosis, the infection is mild and asymptomatic. Mild cases are usually misdiagnosed as colds or upper respiratory tract infections. Amphotericin B or ketoconazole are used to treat the more severe and diagnosed cases. In extreme cases, surgery may be necessary to remove areas of infection from the lungs.

Cold Sores

DEFINITION: Lesions of the oral area, primarily the margin of the lips, which are caused by herpes simplex type 1 virus; also known as *fever blisters* and *herpes labialis*.

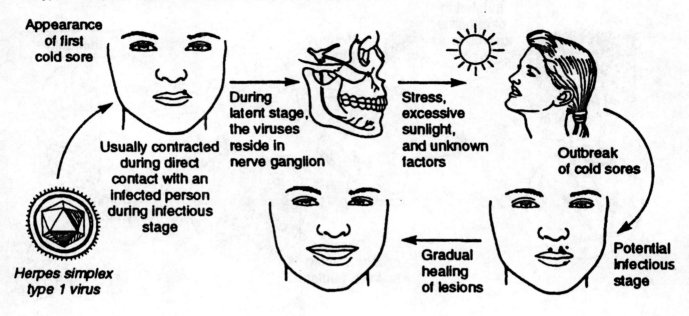

Appearance of first cold sore

Usually contracted during direct contact with an infected person during infectious stage

Herpes simplex type 1 virus

During latent stage, the viruses reside in nerve ganglion

Stress, excessive sunlight, and unknown factors

Outbreak of cold sores

Potential Infectious stage

Gradual healing of lesions

DESCRIPTION: The herpes (Gk. *herpes*, to creep) simplex type 1 virus (HSV-1) contains double-stranded DNA, has an envelope and icosahedral capsid symmetry, replicates in the nucleus, and is about 200 nm in size. It is related to the virus causing genital herpes (HSV-2). HSV-1 is common in the U.S. with an estimated 75% of the population infected with it. During the primary infection, blisters may or may not occur. The virus then migrates to the trigeminal cranial nerve ganglion, where it remains in a latent state. It may again form blisters following trauma, excessive exposure to sunlight, emotional distress, menstruation, fatigue, chronic stress, other respiratory infections, etc. The infectious stage usually occurs when the blisters or sores are apparent. The blisters and lesions usually occur on the lips and occasionally on the gums, tonsils, pharynx, or nose. They require 7 to 10 days to heal.

LABORATORY DIAGNOSIS: HSV-1 can be isolated in cell cultures from vesicular fluid collected from early-stage lesions. Serotyping of the virus isolate to distinguish it from other herpes-group viruses can be done using monoclonal antibodies in immunofluorescence tests.

PREVENTION AND TREATMENT: The best methods of preventing contraction of cold sores are to avoid direct contact (such as kissing a person afflicted with the infectious stage of the virus) and to avoid contact with fomites such as shared eating utensils, hand towels, and toothbrushes. Dental workers and other medical personnel commonly take precautions against infection by using gloves and face shields. A person who has contracted the virus may try to avoid the recurrence of the lesions by avoiding excessive sunlight, managing stress, and generally remaining healthy. Although the disease is untreatable in the latent stage, the drugs acyclovir and foscarnet are somewhat effective in clearing up the lesions.

Colorado Tick Fever

DEFINITION: A relatively benign fever caused by Colorado tick fever virus, and *arbovirus* (arthropod-borne virus) whose vector is the tick, *Dermacentor andersoni*, and whose reservoir is the golden mantle ground squirrel.

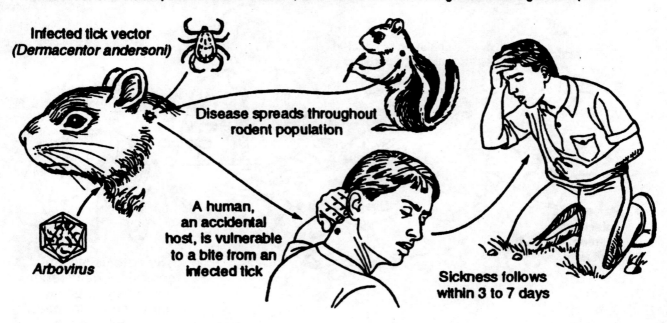

Infected tick vector
(*Dermacentor andersoni*)

Disease spreads throughout rodent population

A human, an accidental host, is vulnerable to a bite from an infected tick

Arbovirus

Sickness follows within 3 to 7 days

DESCRIPTION: The Colorado tick fever virus is interesting in that its genome is segmented consisting of 12 double-stranded RNA molecules. It is classified in the genus *Orbivirus* in the family Reoviridae. Its reservoir in the wild is the golden mantle ground squirrel, with the vector for its transmission to humans being the tick, *Dermacentor andersoni*. The disease is most common among campers in the western United States, particularly those who camp in the Rocky Mountains. The virus gets into the bloodstream and infects erythrocytes during their formation.

SIGNS AND SYMPTOMS: The disease begins with chills and an episode of fever, followed, in about 50% of cases, by another episode of fever a few days later. Other symptoms include headaches, muscle aches, nausea, and general malaise. The recovery time is usually 2–3 weeks, with antibodies persisting in the blood for up to 20 weeks. The mortality rate of Colorado tick fever is low, although infected children are more likely to die than adults.

LABORATORY DIAGNOSIS: Rapid diagnosis is possible by immunofluorescent staining of virus in the patient's erythrocytes. Viruses can be cultured from serum or whole blood by inoculating suckling mice. A diagnostic rise in antibody titer can be shown in acute and convalescent sera using ELISA tests, complement fixation, or serum neutralization tests.

PREVENTION AND TREATMENT: The best method of prevention is to avoid being bitten by ticks when camping or hiking in endemic areas. Wearing protective clothing and using arthropod repellents are advisable. It is also important to inspect clothing and the entire body surface for the presence of ticks following campouts or picnics in locations known to be infested with ticks. Ticks should be removed by grasping them with fine tweezers at the point of attachment to the skin and pulling slowly and steadily. The bite should then be cleansed. Ticks should not be removed with bare hands or by crushing them between the fingers. Treatment of Colorado tick fever is primarily directed to relieving the symptoms of the disease.

Common Cold (also called coryza) Gk. *koryza*, nasal discharge

DEFINITION: A disease of the upper respiratory tract, caused by one of over 200 different viruses, many of which are *rhinoviruses*. Symptoms include nasal stuffiness and discharge, malaise, coughing, and sneezing.

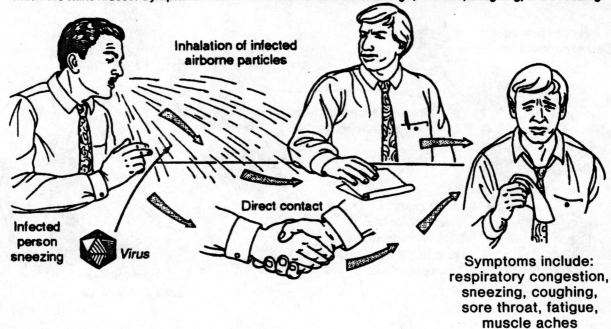

Inhalation of infected airborne particles

Direct contact

Infected person sneezing

Virus

Symptoms include:
respiratory congestion,
sneezing, coughing,
sore throat, fatigue,
muscle aches

DESCRIPTION: The common cold is the most common of infectious diseases, with the average American being ill twice each year. There are over 200 different viruses which may cause the disease. Most of these are grouped within the RNA virus families *Picornaviridae* (including the *rhinoviruses*) or *Coronaviridae*. These viruses reproduce best at temperatures of about 33° C, the temperature of the nasal passages. It is, therefore, usually only the epithelial lining of the respiratory passageways that become infected. Occasionally, an infection secondarily spreads to the paranasal sinuses, inner ear, or lower respiratory tract. An infection usually lasts for about a week, during which time the virus is fought off with IgA antibodies. Colds may be transmitted by the inhalation of infected airborne particles, through direct hand-to-hand contact with an infected person, or through contact with contaminated fomites. Colds occur more frequently during winter months, probably due to decreased resistance and increased contact with infected persons.

SIGNS AND SYMPTOMS: Symptoms of a cold are nasal stuffiness and discharge, sneezing, coughing, and a sore throat. As the disease progresses, nasal discharge changes from clear and runny to yellow and thick.

LABORATORY DIAGNOSIS: Laboratory testing is usually not performed for the diagnosis of common colds.

PREVENTION AND TREATMENT: Frequent hand washing, avoiding contact with infected people and keeping the hands away from the face are the most effective ways of preventing the "catching of a cold." Vaccinations are not available and perhaps would be ineffective because there are so many different serotypes causing infection, and immunity for each lasts a relatively short time. Currently there is no cure for the common cold, although there are a number of medicines available to relieve the symptoms.

Conjunctivitis (kon-jungk-ti-vi'tis)

DEFINITION: Hyperemia, or the presence of an excess of blood, in the conjunctiva of the eye due to infection, allergy, or chemical reactions; commonly known as *pinkeye*.

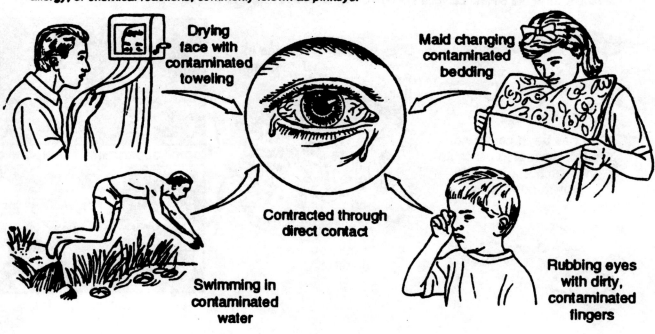

Drying face with contaminated toweling

Maid changing contaminated bedding

Contracted through direct contact

Swimming in contaminated water

Rubbing eyes with dirty, contaminated fingers

DESCRIPTION: Conjunctivitis is considered the most common eye affliction in the Western Hemisphere. Although it is most commonly due to infection with the pseudomonads or adenoviruses, conjunctivitis may also be caused by many other bacterial and viral agents, as well as allergies. Conjunctivitis involves dilation and congestion of the blood vessels of the conjunctiva, the mucous membrane covering the anterior portion of the eyeball and forming the inside membrane lining each eyelid. Infection usually begins in one eye and is often spread to the other. Transmission of the organisms causing conjunctivitis is usually by direct hand-to-hand contact with an infected person. Towels, pillows, contact lenses, microscopes, and other materials which may come in contact with an infected eye are also fomites. Conjunctivitis generally has no permanent effect on vision.

Inclusion conjunctivitis is caused by *Chlamydia trachomatis* which is the leading cause of preventable blindness in the world. It is transmitted by hand-contact, houseflies, and from the infected uterine cervix during birth.

Causative agents, symptoms, and treatment

Causes	Symptoms	Treatment
Bacterial Pseudomonads Streptococcus pneumoniae Staphylococcus aureus Hemophilus influenzae Neisseria gonorrhoeae	Itching, burning, sensation of a foreign body in the eye, eyelids show crust from a sticky discharge	Responds well to topical sulfonamides, or antibiotic therapy
Chlamydia trachomatis	Inclusion conjunctivitis, corneal scarring, blindness	Erythromycin, tetracyclines

Viral
Adenoviruses, poxviruses,
   herpes viruses,
   papovaviruses, myxoviruses
	Mild itching, sensation of a foreign body in the eye, copious tearing, watery discharge	Resists treatment, but broad spectrum antibiotic drops may be used to prevent secondary bacterial invasion

Creutzfeldt-Jakob Disease (CJD)

DEFINITION: A rare, terminal disease in which an undetermined infectious agent causes rapidly progressive degeneration of the central nervous system (CNS); related to kuru and scrapie.

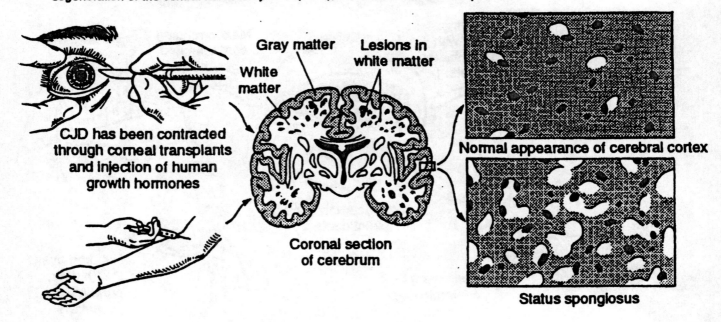

CJD has been contracted through corneal transplants and injection of human growth hormones

White matter

Gray matter

Lesions in white matter

Normal appearance of cerebral cortex

Coronal section of cerebrum

Status spongiosus

DESCRIPTION: Creutzfeldt-Jakob disease (CJD) affects one of every one million people between the ages of 40 and 65. The unidentified agent which causes CJD has been called a *slow virus* or *unconventional virus* because of its unusual resistance to inactivation by heat or radiation, very small size, and long incubation and latency periods. It has been hypothesized that the CJD agent is a very small strand of nucleic acid surrounded by a tightly-packed protein coat which protects it from inactivation, or is a self-replicating protein without nucleic acid called a proteinaceous infectious particle or *prion*. Infection by this agent causes status spongiosus in which brain tissue takes on an uncharacteristic spongy appearance, accompanied by severe loss of neurons, and widespread atrophy of the cerebral cortex. The infection produces no inflammation in the CNS tissue or change in the cerebrospinal fluid and provokes no immune response. The only known means of transmission for CJD is through penetration of the skin by infected tissue. CJD cannot be transmitted by routine contact with body fluids, but has been contracted through corneal transplants, or the injection of cadaveric human growth hormone. Although patient isolation procedures are not necessary, special care should be taken in dealing with CJD patients and in sterilizing contaminated equipment to avoid skin penetration.

SIGNS AND SYMPTOMS: Early stages are characterized by alteration in behavior, memory, and reasoning. The prevalent symptom of CJD is myoclonus, or shock-like muscle contractions, which appear spontaneously or in response to noise or light. Lack of muscle coordination and coherent speech, and an abnormal EEG (brain wave) pattern are other characteristic signs. The disease eventually results in coma and death to the patient within 3 to 24 months after the onset of symptoms.

LABORATORY DIAGNOSIS: A characteristic EEG recording is indicative of CJD diagnosis. Post-mortem histopathologic examination of brain tissue is required for confirmation.

PREVENTION AND TREATMENT: Hospital workers should follow established procedures for the prevention of transmission of blood- and tissue-borne etiologic agents. No effective treatment for CJD is known.

Croup (kroop) A.S. *kropan*, to cry aloud

DEFINITION: Croup refers to a syndrome of childhood respiratory diseases characterized by a barking, resonant cough and difficulty breathing; caused by either viruses or bacteria.

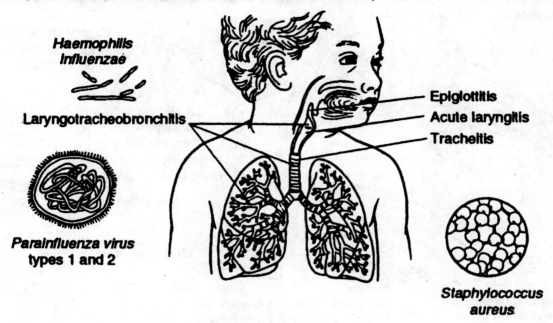

Haemophilis Influenzae

Laryngotracheobronchitis

Parainfluenza virus types 1 and 2

Epiglottitis
Acute laryngitis
Tracheitis

Staphylococcus aureus

DESCRIPTION: The croup diseases usually affect the larynx and upper trachea, causing swelling or obstruction. Croup is most common during the winter months in children ages six months to three years. Viruses and bacteria are the principal agents, though some infections may accompany diphtheria and pertussis. The most serious complication of croup is complete airway obstruction.

SIGNS AND SYMPTOMS: The symptoms of croup are dependent upon the infected region of the respiratory system.

Acute Laryngitis—sudden onset of hoarseness and barking cough that worsen at night. The etiologic agent is unknown. Severe dyspnea generally wakens the child.

Laryngotracheobronchitis—the most common form of croup, characterized by coughing and difficult breathing. It is caused by *parainfluenza virus types 1, 2*, and *3*.

Epiglottitis—caused by the bacterium *Haemophilis influenzae*. This condition can rapidly progress to severe respiratory distress. The child has a "frog-like" croak, a bright red throat and avoids swallowing because it is so painful. The child should be examined quickly before the swollen, infected epiglottis occludes the airway causing asphyxia and death. This condition usually occurs in older children.

Tracheitis—caused by *Staphylococcus aureus*. This condition causes increased fever, and production of thick, purulent tracheal secretions. Suctioning may help to relieve respiratory distress.

LABORATORY DIAGNOSIS: Diagnosis is made by culture of bacteria from respiratory specimens on blood agar and chocolate agar. Parainfluenza viruses are detected in cell culture or by direct immunofluorescence in respiratory specimens.

PREVENTION AND TREATMENT: Early recognition is important in all of these croup syndromes. Endotracheal intubation or tracheostomy may be required of respirations are seriously inhibited. Ampicillin, amoxicillin, and chloramphenicol are administered for the conditions caused by bacteria. Symptomatic treatment includes humidification of the air. Oxygen may also be administered by the use of a face mask. The *H. influenzae* type b (HIB) vaccine should be administered to children at 24 months of age to prevent epiglottitis, meningitis, otitis media, bacteremia, pneumonia, and many other complications of *H. influenzae* infection.

Cryptococcosis (krip"to-kok-o'sis) Gk. *kryptos*, hidden; *kokkos*, berry

DEFINITION: A systemic fungus infection that may involve any organ of the body, including lungs, or skin, but having a predilection for the brain and the meninges. It is caused by the yeast-like organism *Cryptococcus neoformans*; formerly called *torulosis*.

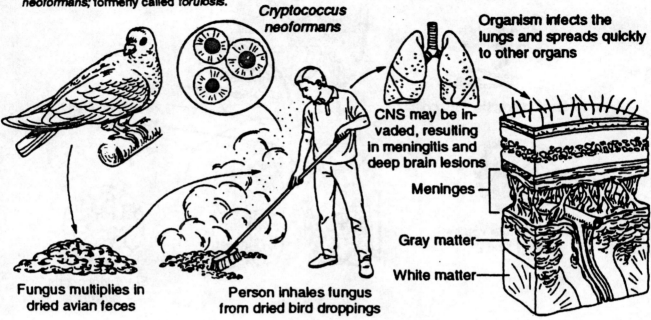

Cryptococcus neoformans

Organism infects the lungs and spreads quickly to other organs

CNS may be invaded, resulting in meningitis and deep brain lesions

Meninges

Gray matter

White matter

Fungus multiplies in dried avian feces

Person inhales fungus from dried bird droppings

DESCRIPTION: The *Cryptococcus neoformans* organism, a budding yeast, is found in avian feces worldwide. The disease may be transmitted when particles from dried, infected bird droppings are inhaled. Birds are not affected, but humans, dogs, cats, cattle, and horses are susceptible. The most significant source of infection for humans is the droppings of the common pigeon. The organism infects the lungs initially, but if the host is debilitated or immunologically impaired, it will spread quickly from the lungs to other organs, particularly the brain where it causes deep lesions in both the gray and white matter. Exudates accumulate on the brain's surface and meningitis is also present. *C. neoformans* is the only encapsulated yeast to invade the CNS.

SIGNS AND SYMPTOMS: Infection can cause the development of single or multiple abscesses in various locations depending on the area of infection. The cerebral type of the disease is characterized by headache, dizziness, vertigo, and extreme stiffness of the neck. In the later stages, coma and respiratory failure occur. This condition is often mistaken for a brain tumor. Cerebral and meningeal forms of cryptococcosis are usually fatal.

LABORATORY DIAGNOSIS: Positive cultures of sputum and cerebrospinal fluid are diagnostic. Negative stains of specimens using India ink or nigrosin examined under high-dry magnification demonstrate the encapsulated organisms. Cryptococcal antigen is found by agglutination of antibody-coated latex particles.

PREVENTION AND TREATMENT: Avoiding large accumulations of bird feces is an important preventative technique. Persons in close contact with many birds should wear a mask when cleaning bird droppings. Amphotericin B has been effective (80 to 90% cure rate) in treating patients infected with cryptococcosis. Other antimicrobial drugs may also be used. Prognosis is poor for AIDS patients with cryptococcosis.

Cystitis (sis-ti'tis) Gk. *kystis*, bladder; *itis*, inflammation

DEFINITION: Inflammation of the urinary bladder usually occurring secondary to lower urinary tract infections. It can be caused by a variety of organisms, of which *Escherichia coli* is the most common.

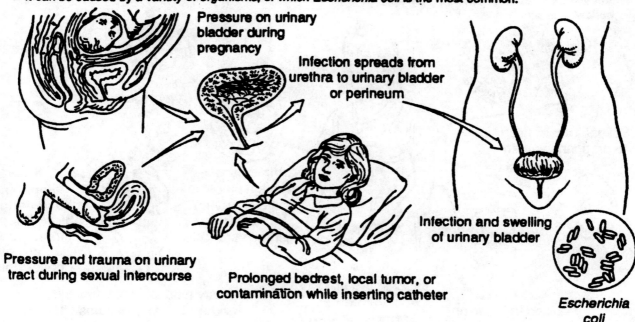

Pressure on urinary bladder during pregnancy

Infection spreads from urethra to urinary bladder or perineum

Pressure and trauma on urinary tract during sexual intercourse

Prolonged bedrest, local tumor, or contamination while inserting catheter

Infection and swelling of urinary bladder

Escherichia coli

DESCRIPTION: Cystitis is a common condition, especially in women. Females experience urinary bladder inflammation 30 times more frequently than males. It is thought that every woman will have cystitis at least once during her lifetime. Predisposing factors for the infection in women are the relatively short urethra (4 cm), pressure and trauma of sexual intercourse, and pregnancy. Risk factors for the infection in both sexes may be local tumors, prolonged bedrest, or the insertion of catheters. Circumcision reduces the risk of cystitis in males. Associated organs such as the ureters, kidneys, and prostate (in males) may also be involved in ascending infections. Organisms, other than *E. coli*, found in cases of cystitis include staphylococci, *Proteus, Klebsiella, Enterobacter, Pseudomonas*, and enterococci.

SIGNS AND SYMPTOMS: Lower abdominal or vaginal pain may be present. Urinary frequency and urgency is also a sign because the urinary bladder loses its elasticity. Urination becomes painful, and pus and blood may be present in the urine.

LABORATORY DIAGNOSIS: The presence of ≥100,000 bacteria per ml of urine is diagnostic of cystitis. The organisms are detected by direct microscopic examination of stained or unstained centrifuged or uncentrifuged urine. Culture techniques are also used. Detection of pyuria (leukocytes in the urine) indicates infection. Direct microscopic examination or the esterase dipstick test detect pyuria.

PREVENTION AND TREATMENT: Careful genital hygiene minimizes the chance of cystitis. To reduce the risk of urinary infections, a female should wipe her anal region in a posterior direction, away from the urethral opening. Ampicillin or sulfa drugs may be given to decrease the risk of ascending kidney disease and to quickly relieve the symptoms. Other definitive therapy will be required if the basic cause of the disease is an obstruction, tumor, or structural defect in the urinary tract.

Cytomegalic Inclusion Disease Gk. *kytos*, cell; *megas*, large

DEFINITION: A severe, often fatal disease of newborns that usually affects the salivary glands, lungs, kidneys, and liver. It is a major cause of neurological birth defects. Infection is from *cytomegalovirus (CMV)* and is worldwide in occurrence.

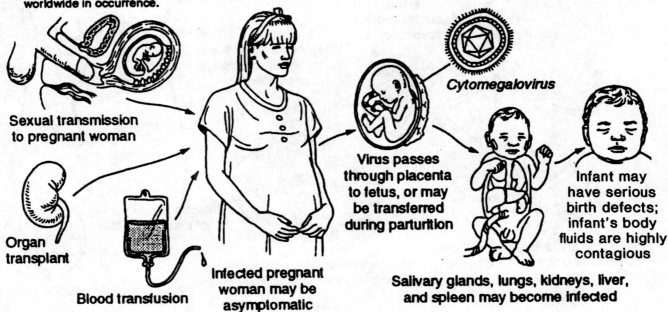

Sexual transmission to pregnant woman

Organ transplant

Blood transfusion

Infected pregnant woman may be asymptomatic

Cytomegalovirus

Virus passes through placenta to fetus, or may be transferred during parturition

Salivary glands, lungs, kidneys, liver, and spleen may become infected

Infant may have serious birth defects; infant's body fluids are highly contagious

DESCRIPTION: The cytomegalovirus (CMV) is one of a group of species-specific herpesviruses. It infects human salivary glands, organs of the respiratory system, kidneys, and liver. Cytomegalic inclusion disease is frequently sexually transmitted. Cytomegaloviruses can readily cross the placenta in a pregnant woman resulting in an infection of the fetal respiratory, digestive, or genital tracts. It may also infect mucous membranes of a baby during parturition. Cytomegalic inclusion disease has a 3–5 week incubation period. Organ transplantation and blood transfusion are additional modes for possible transmission of CMV. CMV is widely distributed throughout the world especially in countries on a lower socioeconomic level. CMV is known to depress both cell-mediated and humoral immune responses which can make the host vulnerable to a superinfection with bacteria or fungi.

SIGNS AND SYMPTOMS: In adults, infection causes acute febrile illness, an enlarged spleen, and an increase in the circulating lymphocytes. Primary infection and re-activation infections are often inapparent. Infants show liver and spleen enlargement and severe jaundice. A congenital infection can produce such serious birth defects as microcephaly, hydrocephaly, blindness, deafness, and mental retardation. CMV is the leading viral cause of birth defects in the U.S. A pregnant mother may be asymptomatic and still be infected, thus transferring the virus to her fetus.

LABORATORY DIAGNOSIS: Previous infections are detected by IgG antibody determinations using ELISA tests; current CMV infections are detected using IgM antibody determinations in ELISA tests and by culture of infectious CMV from blood or urine.

PREVENTION AND TREATMENT: An affected individual actively sheds the virus in body fluids and care should be taken, therefore, when contacting an affected person (e.g., when handling diapers of an affected child). Anti-metabolites or anti-viral agents are frequently used to treat infections. Detecting the presence of CMV is very important especially in pregnant women. Part of the TORCH series of tests for pregnant women includes a test for this infection ("C" in TORCH stands for cytomegalovirus).

Dengue Fever (den'ga)

DEFINITION: Febrile disease caused by a mosquito-borne *flavivirus*; commonly know as *breakbone fever.*

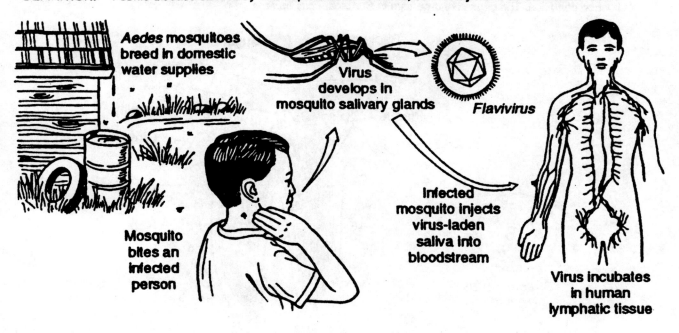

Aedes mosquitoes breed in domestic water supplies

Virus develops in mosquito salivary glands

Flavivirus

Mosquito bites an infected person

Infected mosquito injects virus-laden saliva into bloodstream

Virus incubates in human lymphatic tissue

DESCRIPTION: Dengue fever is caused by an enveloped RNA virus, 45–55 nm in diameter with an icosahedral nucleocapsid. The virus is transmitted among humans by the *Aedes aegypti* mosquito, which lives near human populations and breeds on and around domestic water supplies. After a mosquito feeds on the blood of an infected human, viral particles develop in its salivary glands in 8 to 12 days. When this mosquito bites another human, it injects virus-laden saliva into the bloodstream. Following an incubation period of 3 to 8 days in the human lymphatic tissues, symptoms appear suddenly. While dengue fever is often a relatively mild condition, the disease can progress to the more severe dengue *hemorrhagic fever* (DHF) or even more severe *dengue shock syndrome* (DSS). Although all three conditions are caused by the same virus, they differ significantly. DHF is characterized by increased vascular permeability and altered homeostasis which cause hemorrhage. DHF is almost exclusively Asiatic, and children under 14 are the most frequent victims. The distinguishing symptoms of DSS are hypotension and circulatory failure due to extensive plasma loss. The mortality rate for both DHF and DSS is 5 to 10%.

SIGNS AND SYMPTOMS: Fever reaching 104° F is noted during the first 3 to 6 days of the illness. Muscle and joint pain, headache, retro-orbital pain, and a rash during the 3rd to 5th day are also common symptoms. Signs of subcutaneous bleeding, known as *petechiae,* is an indication of the more serious forms of the disease.

LABORATORY DIAGNOSIS: Diagnosis is made by isolation of virus from patient serum in mosquito cell lines or live mosquitoes. Serologic diagnosis using acute and convalescent sera is the alternative.

PREVENTION AND TREATMENT: The most effective prevention is to reduce and control the *Aedes aegypti* mosquito population. No effective vaccines for the dengue virus are available and no effective treatment for dengue fever is known. Aspirin should be avoided to prevent exacerbation of hemorrhage.

Dental Caries (Tooth Decay)

DEFINITION: Dental caries is the end result of microbial metabolism within dental plaque and is a common childhood condition. The causative organism is *Streptococcus mutans*.

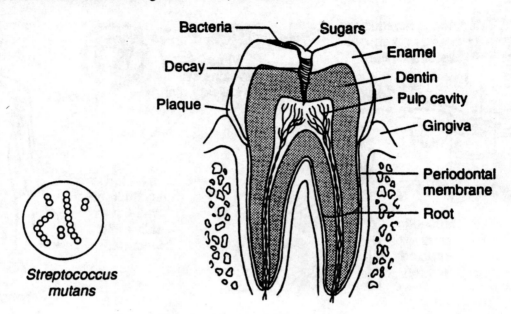

Streptococcus mutans

DESCRIPTION: Dental caries is a wide-spread problem among people living in underdeveloped nations and people who do not practice good dental hygiene. An estimated 80% of the teeth removed from 15–24 year-olds are lost due to caries. *Plaque* is a substance that accumulates on teeth, especially in cracks and fissures, and is generally a promoter for caries. The acid-forming bacteria lodge in the plaque and produce a chemical attack on the durable enamel that covers teeth. Over a period of weeks or months, the cavity extends into the dentin where the bacterial organisms spread more rapidly. Eventually, the lesion penetrates the pulp cavity where an inflammatory response causes the acute pain known as a *toothache*. An untreated, infected tooth will eventually become devitalized as the live cells of the pulp are killed.

SIGNS AND SYMPTOMS: A caries is frequently asymptomatic until the infection reaches the pulp where nerve endings are present. When the cavity becomes this deep, throbbing pain results. The pain of cavities in untreated teeth is an important cause of inattention in children.

PREVENTION AND TREATMENT: Responsible dental hygiene, including the regular use of dental floss is an important deterrent to dental caries. A healthy diet and the avoidance of eating high sucrose snacks between meals are also important. Sugar supplies nutrients for increased bacterial growth. Dentists treat caries of enamel and dentin by removing affected material and replacing it with a hard material filling. Caries may, however, reactivate around the borders of the filling. Currently, most dentists use a sealant as a form of prevention to cover the teeth before caries develop. Fluoride added to culinary water and toothpaste works to harden the enamel and further prevent caries.

Diphtheria (dip-the're-a) Gk. *diphthera*, membrane

DEFINITION: An acute infectious respiratory disease caused by the exotoxin of *Corynebacterium diphtheriae*, a pleomorphic gram-positive rod. It is characterized by the presence of a grayish pseudomembranous growth in the throat, or nasopharynx.

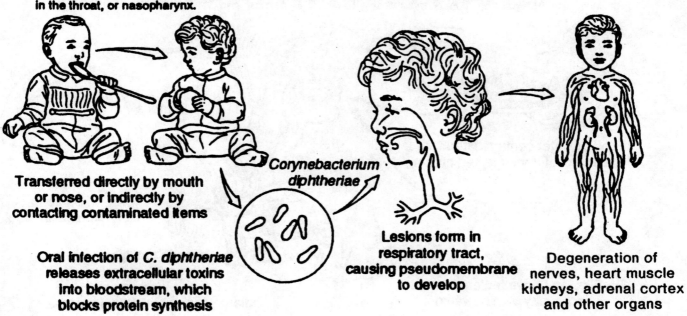

Transferred directly by mouth or nose, or indirectly by contacting contaminated items

Corynebacterium diphtheriae

Oral infection of *C. diphtheriae* releases extracellular toxins into bloodstream, which blocks protein synthesis

Lesions form in respiratory tract, causing pseudomembrane to develop

Degeneration of nerves, heart muscle kidneys, adrenal cortex and other organs

DESCRIPTION: Diphtheria is an upper respiratory tract infection that is most common in children. It is transferred directly by drops expelled from the mouth and nose of infected persons, or indirectly via contaminated toys, dishes, and other fomites. After exposure and growth of the organisms in the nasopharynx, the exotoxin is released into the bloodstream and travels throughout the body. Its primary action is to block the synthesis of proteins which leads to cellular injury and degeneration of organs. The sites most frequently affected are nerves, heart muscle, kidneys, and adrenal cortex. Although most carriers harbor bacilli only a short time, a few harbor them permanently even with intensive treatment.

SIGNS AND SYMPTOMS: The first symptoms are a low grade fever and a mild sore throat. Then the initial lesion begins usually on the tonsils, pharynx, larynx, or in the nasal passages. A grayish pseudomembrane appears over the mucosa layer which becomes leathery and may extend down into the trachea or up into the nose. This membrane is a result of the reaction of the cells to the exotoxin. Death can eventually occur from cardiac failure, asphyxiation, or respiratory paralysis.

LABORATORY DIAGNOSIS: Swabs from nasal passages and pharynx should be cultured on Loeffler's slants, tellurite agar, and blood agar. All clinical isolates of *C. diphtheriae* should be tested for toxigenicity by the Elek test.

PREVENTION AND TREATMENT: Children should be immunized at 8 weeks, 4 months, 6 months and 15 months of age with the trivalent diphtheria-pertussis-tetanus (DPT) vaccine. Newborns receive passive immunity through the placenta if the mother is immune. *C. diphtheriae* is easily destroyed by heat (one minute in boiling water) and by chemical disinfectants. Patients with the disease should be isolated and contaminated objects disinfected. Antitoxin may be used for treatment supplemented with anti-microbial therapy (penicillin or erythromycin). Prior to administering the antitoxin, a patient must be tested for hypersensitivity to horse serum.

Dysentery (dis'en-ter''e) Gk. *dys*, painful; *enteron*, intestine

DEFINITION: A digestive tract disorder characterized by frequent, painful passage of low volume stools (diarrhea) containing blood and mucus. Bacillary dysentery is caused primarily by four species of the non-motile, gram-negative *Shigella* bacillus; *S. dysenteriae, S. boydii, S. flexneri,* and *S. sonnei.*

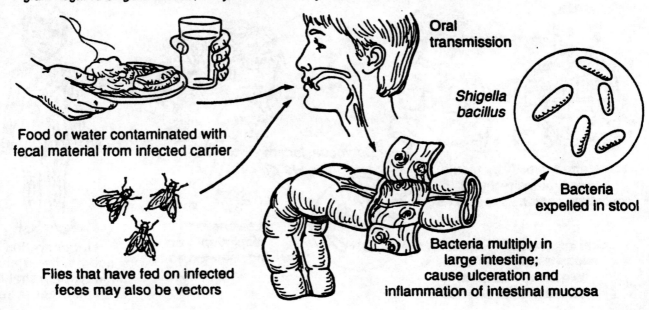

Food or water contaminated with fecal material from infected carrier

Flies that have fed on infected feces may also be vectors

Oral transmission

Shigella bacillus

Bacteria expelled in stool

Bacteria multiply in large intestine; cause ulceration and inflammation of intestinal mucosa

---

DESCRIPTION: Dysentery is caused by many bacterial agents. The *Shigella* bacillus is one of the more virulent of them. Transmission of the pathogens occurs orally through feces-contaminated food, water, or dirty fingers placed in the mouth. Flies are also a common vector. Bacteria grow in the large intestine and cause mucosal ulceration and inflammation. Virulent shigellae produce exotoxins that inhibit protein synthesis, thereby killing cells. Dysentery may occur sporadically or in epidemics. An estimated one third of pediatric deaths in developing countries are attributed to dysentery, diarrhea and resulting dehydration. Humans are the only known reservoir for the *Shigella* bacillus.

SIGNS AND SYMPTOMS: Abdominal pain, fever, cramping, and diarrhea with the passage of bloody mucus are the primary symptoms. Secondary symptoms include severe dehydration (especially infants) and toxemia.

LABORATORY DIAGNOSIS: Definitive diagnosis of bacillary dysentery depends on the isolation of shigellae by selective media. Appropriate culture media include blood, desoxycholate, and Salmonella-Shigella (S-S) agars. Differential diagnosis is made by placing a drop of methylene blue—stained stool sample on a microscope slide. The presence of abundant neutrophils helps in distinguishing shigellosis from diarrheal syndromes caused by viruses and enterotoxigenic bacteria. Amebic dysentery is excluded by the absence of trophozoites.

PREVENTION AND TREATMENT: Prevention techniques include practicing good sanitation, consumption of only properly prepared food, and drinking only purified water. In a healthy adult, dysentery generally resolves spontaneously in about a week. In debilitated adults or small children, dysentery may be life threatening. Fluid and electrolyte replacement is important therapy. Infection may provide some degree of immunity, but the same person may also have two episodes in a single season. A preventative vaccination is not currently available. Tetracycline, chloramphenicol, and ampicillin can all be used on susceptible bacterial strains. However, *Shigella* has resistance transfer factors which have given some strains worldwide resistance to antibiotic therapy

Encephalitis (en-sef"a-li'tis) Gk. *enkephalos*, brain; *itis*, inflammation

DEFINITION: Inflammation of the brain accompanied by degenerative changes. Encephalitis may be due to a primary viral infection of the brain, bacterial or parasitic infections, or result from immunologic reactions to chronic or preexisting infections; also called *brain fever.*

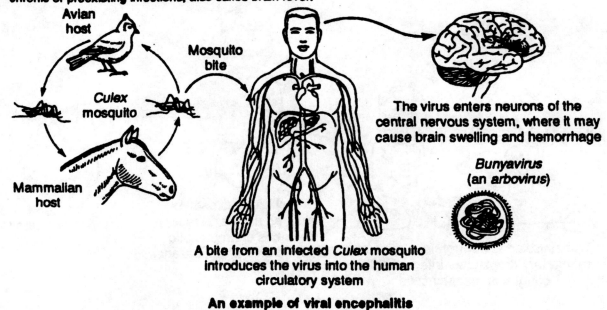

Avian host

Mosquito bite

Culex mosquito

Mammalian host

The virus enters neurons of the central nervous system, where it may cause brain swelling and hemorrhage

Bunyavirus (an *arbovirus*)

A bite from an infected *Culex* mosquito introduces the virus into the human circulatory system

An example of viral encephalitis

DESCRIPTION: Viral infection may cause primary or post-infectious encephalitis. *Primary encephalitis* results from direct viral infection of the brain. Arbo-, polio-, echo-, and coxsackie viruses can cause epidemic encephalitis, while herpes simplex and herpes zoster viruses may result in sporadic cases of encephalitis. Primary encephalitis can show signs of aseptic meningitis (CSF with normal glucose, elevated number of lymphocytes, and absence of bacteria) and the causative virus may frequently be identified in the CSF. *Post-infectious (para-infectious or allergic) encephalitis* is an immunological complication of a viral infection and represents the majority of cases of encephalitis. Viral infections resulting in cases of post-infectious encephalitis include measles, chicken pox, and rubella. The immune reaction to the infection usually develops in 5 to 10 days and causes a progressive perivascular neural demyelination. Findings of aseptic meningitis are usually absent in post-infectious encephalitis and the causative virus is never identified in the CSF.

Some arbovirus-caused encephalitides are transmitted by insect vectors, mosquitoes of the genus *Culex* being the most important. The virus is injected into the blood or lymph of the host and then enters neurons of the brain. Large mammals and birds are the principal hosts, and humans are generally considered accidental hosts. Other infection causing encephalitis include leptospirosis, toxoplasmosis, trichinosis, syphilis, tuberculosis, mycoplasma infections, and others.

SIGNS AND SYMPTOMS: Encephalitis, which may include symptoms of meningitis (fever, headache, stiff neck, nausea, and vomiting), is characterized by cerebral dysfunction: alteration in consciousness, personality changes, seizures, cranial nerve abnormalities, paralysis, and paresis. The extent of symptoms varies considerably.

PREVENTION AND TREATMENT: Prevention measures include vaccination (where appropriate vaccines exist) avoidance of transmission of the infectious agent, and controlling the population of insect vectors (such as spraying to kill mosquitoes). No effective antiviral agent is available for most forms of viral encephalitis. An exception is herpes simplex encephalitis which may be controlled if treated early with vidarabine or acyclovir. Patients with encephalitis may experience permanent nervous system damage.

Erythema Infectiosum Gk. *erythema*, redness

DEFINITION: A contagious form of erythema that is manifested by rose-colored eruptions. It generally occurs in epidemics and is caused by the *human parvovirus B 19;* also called *Fifth disease,* or *slapped cheek syndrome.*

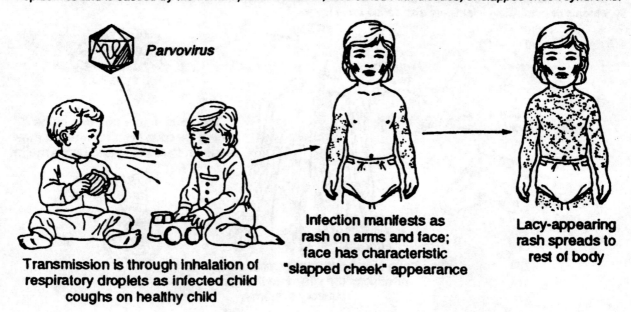

Parvovirus

Transmission is through inhalation of respiratory droplets as infected child coughs on healthy child

Infection manifests as rash on arms and face; face has characteristic "slapped cheek" appearance

Lacy-appearing rash spreads to rest of body

DESCRIPTION: Erythema infectiosum is a mild, viral disease which affects primarily children, but in a large epidemic many cases are also seen in adults. It is a fairly common condition that is transmitted through the respiratory secretions from infected persons. The causative agent is the *human parvovirus B 19.* This infection causes aplastic crisis in patients with hemolytic anemia and in children who are homozygous for sickle cell disease. Erythema infectiosum has an incubation period that varies from one to seven weeks. Lifelong immunity follows infection.

SIGNS AND SYMPTOMS: The prodomal stage in children lasts 2–4 days and is accompanied by low grade fever and occasionally joint pains. When the red, macular rash develops, it begins on the arms and face and then spreads to the body. The rash appears reticular or mesh-like on the body, while the face has a "slapped-cheek" appearance. The rash lasts approximately one week. In adults, the rash on the face is less conspicuous. Joint complaints are also more common in adults, and itching is present.

Some evidence suggests an association between infection during pregnancy and congenital defects in the fetus. *Hydrops fetalis* may occur as well as a variable pattern of residual defects. Spontaneous abortions may also occur as a result of fetal death.

LABORATORY DIAGNOSIS: Laboratory procedures are not widely available for the diagnosis of erythema infectiosum, however, some laboratories employ ELISA or RIA tests for the detection of specific IgM antibodies or high titers of IgG antibodies. The virus is not readily culturable, but viral antigens can be detected by RIA or viral nucleic acids with specific DNA probes.

PREVENTION AND TREATMENT: No specific treatment is available. The signs and symptoms disappear spontaneously. This condition must be differentiated from measles and other viral infections which manifest a rash. Pregnant women should avoid contact with persons suffering from acute erythema infectiosum.

Food Poisoning

DEFINITION: Food poisoning is a broad term referring to illnesses acquired by the ingestion of infected foods which are most often improperly prepared. *Food intoxications* are caused by ingestion of pre-formed toxins, while *food borne infections* result from ingestion of organisms growing in the food.

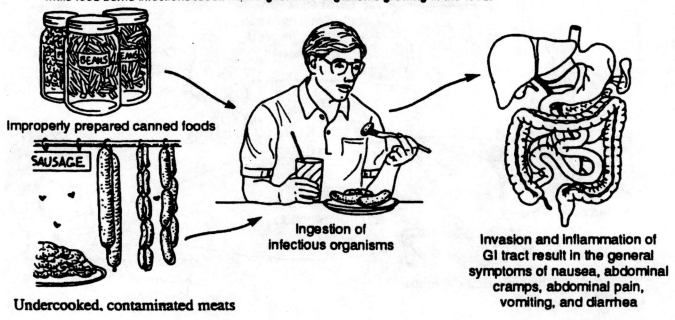

Improperly prepared canned foods

Undercooked, contaminated meats

Ingestion of infectious organisms

Invasion and inflammation of GI tract result in the general symptoms of nausea, abdominal cramps, abdominal pain, vomiting, and diarrhea

DESCRIPTION: Several pathogens causing food poisoning are listed in order of prevalence.

	Cause of disease	Pathogenic mechanism	Foods
S. aureus	Ingestion of preformed toxin	Enterotoxins	High protein foods: meats and dairy products; sauces and salads
Salmonella	Ingestion of infectious organism	Mucosal invasion	Poultry, eggs
Shigella	Ingestion of infectious organism	Mucosal invasion, exotoxins	Various foods
E. coli	Ingestion of infectious organism	Enterotoxins, mucosal invasion	Food prepared with contaminated water, uncooked vegetables
C. botulinum	Ingestion of preformed toxin	Exotoxin	Canned vegetables, meats
C. perfringens	Ingestion of infectious organism	Exotoxin released in GI tract	Meats, poultry

SIGNS AND SYMPTOMS: The symptoms of food poisoning by a particular pathogen are essentially the same as a gastrointestinal infection with the same pathogen. Ingestion of a preformed toxin usually results in a more rapid onset of symptoms. Diagnosis includes bacteriologic culture of stool and left-over food.

	Illness	Incubation	Symptoms
S. aureus	Gastroenteritis	1–6 hrs.	Vomiting, abdominal cramps, diarrhea
Salmonella	Dysentery	6–48 hrs.	Nausea, vomiting, watery diarrhea
Shigella	Dysentery	6–48 hrs.	Cramping, bloody diarrhea, fever
E. coli	Traveler's diarrhea	6–48 hrs.	Watery diarrhea
C. botulinum	Botulism	12–36 hrs.	Headache, blurred vision, muscle weakness, paralysis
C. perfringens	Food poisoning	8–24 hrs.	Nausea, watery diarrhea, abdominal pain

PREVENTION AND TREATMENT: Food poisoning results when foods carrying the infectious organisms are improperly prepared. Proper handling, cooking, or preserving of food eliminates the risk of food poisoning. Treatment of food poisoning includes administering appropriate antitoxins and antibiotics, and restoration of fluid and electrolyte balance.

Foot and Mouth Disease

DEFINITION: A viral disease primarily affecting ungulates (hoofed mammals) that is rarely transmitted to humans; caused by foot and mouth disease virus, a *Picornavirus*.

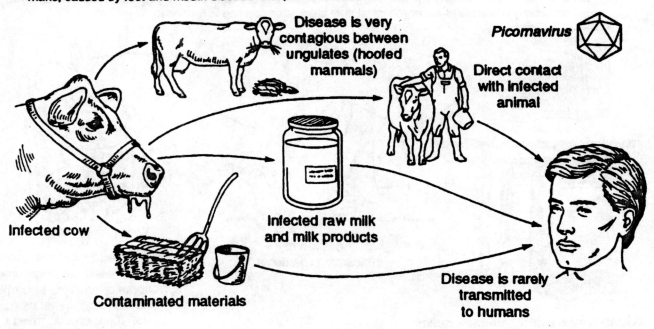

DESCRIPTION: Foot and mouth disease (FMD) is transmitted between animals by direct contact or indirectly by contamination of fodder (feed) with infectious nasal and salivary discharge. Except in Australia, Japan, Britain, and North America, FMD is distributed worldwide and is one of the most contagious of all diseases. FMD may be transmitted to humans by contact with infected animals or by drinking raw (unpasteurized) milk from infected animals. Cattle, sheep, swine, and goats are the animals affected most often, causing this disease to be of great economic concern.

SIGNS AND SYMPTOMS: In animals, the disease is characterized by fever, increased salivation, and the formation of vesicles in the mouth, udder, and on the skin about the hoofs. Humans experience fever, headache and malaise with dryness and burning sensation of the mouth. Vesicles develop on the lips, tongue, mouth, palms, and soles.

LABORATORY DIAGNOSIS: Diagnosis is made by isolation of FMD virus, an acid-sensitive virus, from animal specimens in appropriate host cells. The isolate should be typed to determine to which of the seven immunotypes it belongs.

PREVENTION AND TREATMENT: Vaccination of animals against FMD is done using either the inactivated vaccine or, more recently, a recombinant vaccine. The treatment for infected humans is basically symptomatic because there is no specific treatment against the disease itself. Full recovery usually occurs in 2–3 weeks. Exposed animals should be slaughtered and their bodies should be buried or cremated. The pens of infected animals should be disinfected so the disease will not continue to be transferred. Strict quarantine and importation regulation by government agencies have eliminated FMD in the U.S.

Furuncles and Carbuncles L. *furunculus*, a boil; *carbunculus*, small ember

DEFINITION: Both furuncles and carbuncles are terms for painful abscesses of the skin; usually caused by *staphylococci* bacteria.

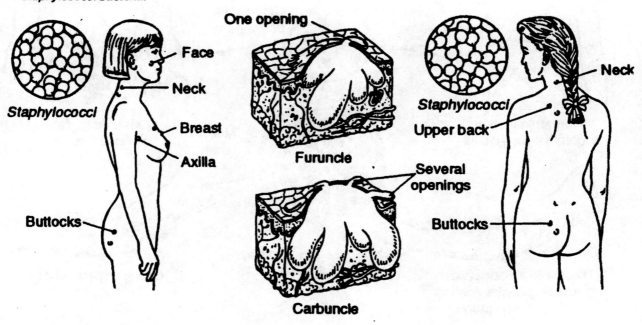

DESCRIPTION: Furuncles are abscesses located in the dermis and subcutaneous tissues of the skin, often called boils. They eventually lead to suppuration and necrosis. The condition of generalized boils is termed *furunculosis*. A lesion that enlarges and develops multiple drainage points is a *carbuncle*. Furuncles and carbuncles often occur in poorly nourished persons and frequently complicate diabetes. These infections may also be spread by direct contact, such as experienced by wrestlers, as the bacteria are transmitted from one person to another through micro-abrasions of the skin.

SIGNS AND SYMPTOMS: Furuncles appear on the neck, axillae, face, buttocks, and breasts. A boil begins in a hair follicle and becomes a smooth and shiny, painful swelling. When a boil ruptures, either spontaneously or after incision, pus is discharged and healing begins. A carbuncle is a painful node that eventually becomes thin and discharges pus through several openings. Carbuncles can enlarge to a size of several centimeters in diameter. Fever, leukocytosis, and sometimes prostration may accompany the carbuncles. Carbuncles usually occur on the neck, upper back, and buttocks.

LABORATORY DIAGNOSIS: Specimen material collected from a lesion cultured on blood agar may grow staphylococci. Sensitivity testing on the isolate should be performed to select an effective antibiotic for treatment.

PREVENTION AND TREATMENT: Antibiotics are generally effective in killing the *staphylococci*. The infected area should be kept covered with warm compresses to promote blood flow. An incision may be necessary to drain the boil. Careful personal and family hygiene should be practiced to avoid contact-spread of the pathogens. Family members should not share towels or washcloths. A boil should not be squeezed as it may rupture and spread into the surrounding subcutaneous tissue. Aseptic techniques should always be used when changing wound dressings on affected areas.

Gangrene (gang'gren) Gk. *gangraina,* an eating sore

DEFINITION: Death of tissue associated with loss of blood supply; often followed by bacterial invasion and putrefaction.

Contamination at abdominal surgical site

Clostridium perfringens

Muscle fiber

Moist gangrene of abdominal wall

Trauma to an appendage permitting contamination at an open wound

Gas between muscle fibers

Gas gangrene of arm

DESCRIPTION: Gangrene may occur in a devitalized tissue and in a wound where there is tissue damage and a reduced supply of oxygen, permitting growth of the invading microorganisms. The infection commonly begins as a mixed infection of aerobes and anaerobes. The aerobes decrease tissue oxygen levels even further creating anaerobic conditions for growth of several species of clostridia, the most important being Clostridium *perfringens.* Gangrene spreads to adjacent tissue, generally affecting extremities or internal organs where it causes massive tissue damage. Gas gangrene is characterized by the appearance of gas pockets produced secondary to the bacterial fermentation of glucose. In moist gangrene, the afflicted area is swollen, moist, and necrotic. The microorganisms may also liberate potent toxins into the bloodstream producing systemic effects.

   Wounds that are most likely to become gangrenous are crushing wounds that result in devitalization of large sections of tissue, especially those that are contaminated with soil (clostridia are found in soil). Wounds received in automobile accidents and war wounds frequently fit into those of high risk for gangrene.

SIGNS AND SYMPTOMS: There is an acute onset with an early sense of increasing weight of the involved area. This is followed by extreme localized pain. The site is swollen, cold, and a foul odor is present. The patient may be nauseous, pale, sweaty, and delirious or apathetic. Septic shock may occur at any time. Gas gangrene is characterized by gas bubbles developing between muscle fibers and a sero-sanguinous discharge. Moist gangrene presents hot, red, and swollen tissue with no pulse present at the afflicted site.

LABORATORY DIAGNOSIS: A gram stain of exudate may show a polymorphic array of organisms. Aerobic culture may be negative while clostridia are isolated in anaerobic culture.

PREVENTION AND TREATMENT: Proper surgical care of a wound, debridement of necrotic tissue, and keeping it clean and sterile is essential. Penicillin and other antibiotics are used to control spreading of the infection but surgical removal of the affected tissue and adjacent regions (amputation) may be necessary. Aerobic conditions should be restored by opening the wound or treating the patient in a hyperbaric chamber in extreme cases.

Genital Herpes (her'pez) Gk. *herpes*, creeping skin disease

DEFINITION: A sexually transmitted disease of the external genitalia and anorectal skin and mucosa; caused by both *Herpes simplex type I virus* and *Herpes simplex type II virus.*

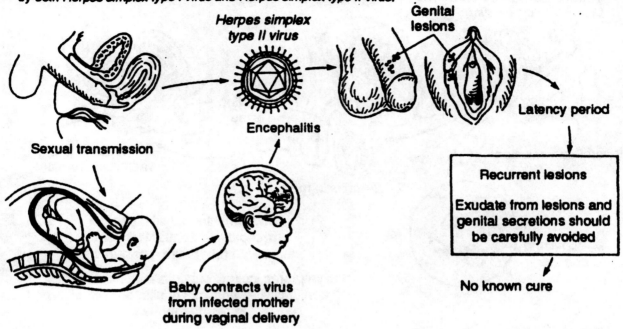

DESCRIPTION: Genital herpes is usually transmitted sexually from patients who have infectious genital lesions or are shedding viruses from asymptomatic sites. After primary infection, the herpes virus may exist in the body as a latent infection in the sacral nerve ganglion and the virus is periodically reactivated. The reactivation often accompanies febrile illness, exposure to cold, sunlight, fatigue, menstruation, or mental strain. One serious complication of genital herpes is that the disease can be transmitted to a fetus during delivery. It may be fatal to the baby. Even if the child does not die, herpetic lesions may be found in all organs including the brain (herpes encephalitis). A cesarean section is usually indicated if a pregnant woman has genital herpes and is infectious with lesions at or near term.

SIGNS AND SYMPTOMS: Itching and soreness are usually present before a small patch of erythema develops. Then a vesicle appears that erodes the tissue. These vesicles are usually painful and heal in about 10 days. They may appear in any part of the genitalia. Usually reactivation episodes heal faster and manifest with fewer blisters. People with recurrent disease can usually expect from 1 to 12 episodes per year, generally decreasing in intensity and frequency with time.

LABORATORY DIAGNOSIS: Diagnosis is made by virus isolation. Vesicular fluid, vaginal and cervical specimens, or cerebrospinal fluid are cultured by standard culture techniques or rapid culture methods. Presumptive identification of HSV is made by observation of a cytopathic effect in cultured cells and confirmed by immuno-staining. The Tzanck test and serology are of little value.

PREVENTION AND TREATMENT: The exudates from lesions and genital secretions should be carefully avoided to prevent transmission of genital herpes. There is no known cure for this infection. Careful partner choice for sexual activity and the use of condoms may reduce the chance of infection. Acyclovir has been of considerable benefit in treating the primary infection and generalized infections. Genital herpes is one of the main factors why cesarean sections are so much more common today. Previous infection with oral HSV type I virus does not provide significant resistance to genital infection with HSV type II virus.

Genital Mycoplasmas Gk. *mykos*, fungus; L. *plasma*, form, mold

DEFINITION: Mycoplasmas refer to several bacteria of the genera *Mycoplasma* and *Ureaplasma;* they are organisms lacking cell walls. The most well known genital mycoplasmas are *Mycoplasma hominis* and *Ureaplasma urealyticum.*

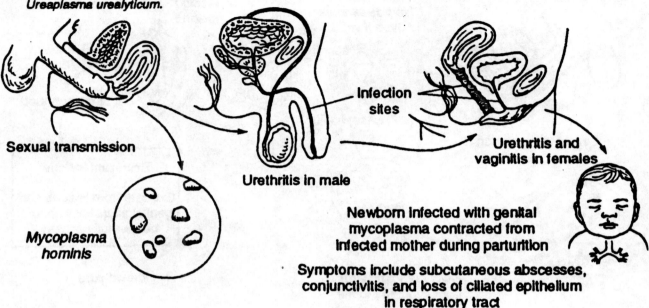

Sexual transmission

Mycoplasma hominis

Urethritis in male

Infection sites

Urethritis and vaginitis in females

Newborn infected with genital mycoplasma contracted from infected mother during parturition

Symptoms include subcutaneous abscesses, conjunctivitis, and loss of ciliated epithelium in respiratory tract

DESCRIPTION: Mycoplasmas are common bacteria in the genital tracts of sexually active males and females. Colonization is related to sexual experience, and females are more readily colonized than are males. The infection can contribute to both male and female infertility, and premature birth if a woman becomes pregnant. *Ureaplasma* has been isolated from the products of conception of patients with repeated spontaneous abortions. Mycoplasmas are most frequent in sexually active persons from lower socioeconomic groups.

SIGNS AND SYMPTOMS: Patients infected with mycoplasma bacteria exhibit inflammatory disease of the reproductive tract and accessory glands, including the urethra and prostate gland in males, and the vagina, cervix, and upper urinary tract in females. In many cases, patients with genital mycoplasmas also suffer from urethritis. Urination becomes more frequent and painful, and a reddening of the mucosa is evident.

LABORATORY DIAGNOSIS: Diagnosis can be made by culture of organisms from appropriate specimen material. An initial rapid screen can be performed in liquid culture media. Growth of typical mycoplasma colonies on semi-solid media is also performed.

PREVENTION AND TREATMENT: Sexual fidelity and the proper use of condoms may minimize the risk of contracting genital mycoplasmas. Spectinomycin and the tetracyclines are effective against the mycoplasmas. Tetracycline is used more often because it is also effective against genital *Chlamydia* infections.

Giardiasis (ji-ar-di'ah-sis) from Alfred Giard, French biologist, 1846–1908

DEFINITION: An infection in the small intestine caused by a population of the protozoan *Giardia lamblia*, giving rise to intestinal cramping and diarrhetic or dysenteric symptoms.

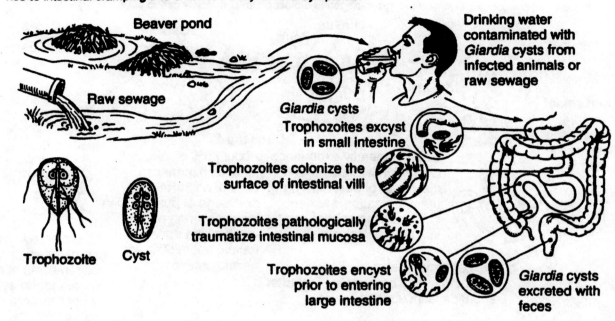

DESCRIPTION: Giardiasis is contracted by drinking water contaminated with cysts from the protozoan *Giardia lamblia*. Once ingested, *trophozoites* excyst (stimulated by stomach acid), then infest the small intestine where they attach to the mucosa of the villi. Because many wild animals, including beaver, are hosts for giardiasis, it may be contracted by backpackers drinking water in wilderness areas. *G. lamblia* is distributed worldwide and is estimated to be carried by 4% to 7% of adults, making it the most frequently identified intestinal parasite found in stool specimens examined in the U.S. public health laboratories. *G. lamblia* is a binucleated, flagellated protozoan that has slow, erratic motility. The *cysts* are ovoid, 8 μm by 12 μm, and contain four nuclei.

SIGNS AND SYMPTOMS: An infection in an adult may be asymptomatic to serious. Giardiasis in children, however, is generally severe and may be life-threatening. An infected person feels nauseous and experiences gastrointestinal cramps. This is accompanied by diarrhea and foul-smelling flatus (gas).

LABORATORY DIAGNOSIS: Diagnosis of giardiasis is made by identification of the cysts in the feces by microscopic examination.

PREVENTION AND TREATMENT: Proper treatment of drinking water (boiling stream water) protects against giardiasis. Because the cyst stage of *G. lamblia* is insensitive to chlorine, filtration of municipal water is necessary. The drugs quinacrine and metronidazole are effective in treating giardiasis.

Gonorrhea (gon"o-re'ah) Gk. *gono*, offspring; *rhoia*, a flow

DEFINITION: An acute infectious sexually transmitted disease of the mucous membranes of the urethra, urinary bladder, cervix, rectum, pharynx, and conjunctiva of the eye; caused by the bacterium *Neisseria gonorrhoeae* or gonococcus, and aerobic, gram-negative diplococcus; commonly called *clap*.

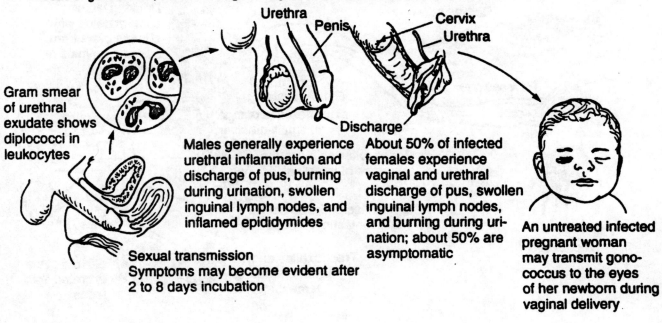

Gram smear of urethral exudate shows diplococci in leukocytes

Urethra
Penis
Cervix
Urethra
Discharge

Males generally experience urethral inflammation and discharge of pus, burning during urination, swollen inguinal lymph nodes, and inflamed epididymides

Sexual transmission
Symptoms may become evident after 2 to 8 days incubation

About 50% of infected females experience vaginal and urethral discharge of pus, swollen inguinal lymph nodes, and burning during urination; about 50% are asymptomatic

An untreated infected pregnant woman may transmit gonococcus to the eyes of her newborn during vaginal delivery.

DESCRIPTION: Gonorrhea is a common sexually transmitted disease. The gonococci attach to mucosal cells by means of pili. Some of them penetrate through mucosal cells to the intracellular spaces and subepithelial tissue where the host's defenses have limited effect on the bacteria. Transmission of gonorrhea to the mucosa of the pharynx is possible during oral-genital contact. Transmission by fomites is uncommon. The incubation period is generally 2 to 8 days. A pregnant woman with gonorrhea who is not treated may transmit the disease to the eyes of her child during delivery.

SIGNS AND SYMPTOMS: Males with gonorrhea suffer inflammation of the urethra, accompanied by painful urination characterized as a burning sensation. Frequently, there is a urethral discharge of yellow, creamy pus, and the inguinal lymph nodes become swollen and tender. If untreated, gonorrhea may spread to the epididymides causing inflammation and scarring of epithelial tissue, and eventual sterility. Symptoms at this stage include sharp and frequent testicular pain. In females, the gonococcus invades the mucosal cells of the urethra and cervix. Symptoms may include a burning sensation during urination, abdominopelvic pain, and some discharge of pus from the urethral and vaginal openings. Salpingitis may occur as a complication and may cause sterility. About 50% of infected women are asymptomatic and unsuspecting carriers of the disease.

LABORATORY DIAGNOSIS: Diagnosis is made by gram stain of the urethral discharge of males and culture of the bacterium from both males and females. Cultures should be on chocolate agar or modified Thayer-Martin medium. Many strains grow best under an atmosphere of 3 to 10% CO_2.

PREVENTION AND TREATMENT: Gonorrhea is the most prevalent sexually transmitted disease in the U.S., with approximately one million reported cases annually. There is no available vaccine. The best prevention is avoidance of sexual promiscuity. Careful use of condoms will reduce the risk. Penicillin-resistant strains of gonococcus are now common. Drug treatment is with *penicillin G* plus *probenecid*, *ampicillim* plus *probenecid*, *tetracycline*, *ceftriaxone*, or *spectinomycin*.

DEFINITION: A contagious and chronic bacterial disease that affects the skin and mucous membranes of the genital, inguinal, and anal regions. It is caused by *Calymmatobacterium granulomatis*, a gram-negative, encapsulated pleomorphic bacterium.

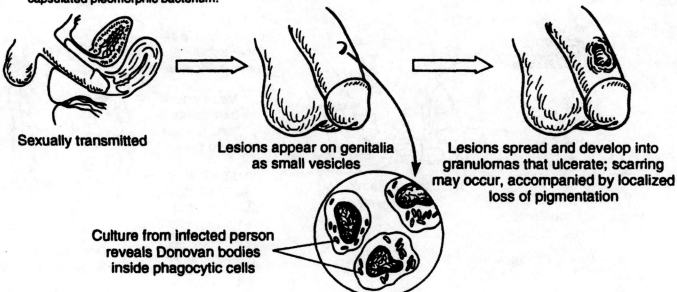

Sexually transmitted

Lesions appear on genitalia as small vesicles

Lesions spread and develop into granulomas that ulcerate; scarring may occur, accompanied by localized loss of pigmentation

Culture from infected person reveals Donovan bodies inside phagocytic cells

DESCRIPTION: Also called donovanosis, granuloma inguinale is a sexually transmitted disease that causes ulceration of the skin and tissues of the groin, anus, and external genitalia. The diagnostic infected cell of granuloma inguinale is a mononuclear phagocyte containing encapsulated rodlike bodies, known as *Donovan bodies*, that have a unique "safety pin" appearance. These cells are stained with Wright's stain or Giemsa stain. Granuloma inguinale is endemic to tropical and subtropical areas and rare in industrialized countries. There is a high incidence of granuloma inguinale in Africa and also a high incidence of heterosexually transmitted human immunodeficiency virus (HIV). It has been suggested that pre-existing granuloma inguinale may be a predisposing factor for AIDS transmission in Africa.

SIGNS AND SYMPTOMS: The initial lesion is a small nodule, vesicle, or papule. It slowly spreads and develops into a large granuloma that ulcerates and may form scars. If the condition is untreated, extensive destruction of the genital organs may occur.

PREVENTION AND TREATMENT: As a sexually transmitted disease, granuloma inguinale is only mildly infectious. Risk factors include promiscuity and pre-existing sexually transmitted diseases. Careful partner choice for sexual activity and the use of condoms will further reduce the chance of infection. Tetracycline, trimethoprim-sulfamethoxazole, and chloramphenicol are all effective medications against the bacterium *C. granulomatis*.

Hepatitis A Gk. *hepatos*, liver; *itis*, inflammation

DEFINITION: Inflammation of the liver caused by the *hepatitis A virus* (HAV); also known as *infectious hepatitis, epidemic hepatitis,* or *short incubation hepatitis.*

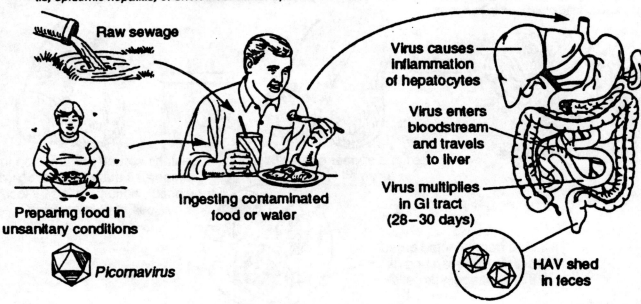

Raw sewage

Preparing food in unsanitary conditions

Picornavirus

Ingesting contaminated food or water

Virus causes inflammation of hepatocytes

Virus enters bloodstream and travels to liver

Virus multiplies in GI tract (28–30 days)

HAV shed in feces

DESCRIPTION: The virus which causes hepatitis A is a single-stranded RNA *picornavirus,* 27 nm in diameter. HAV is shed in the stool of infected patients, making the fecal-oral route the most common means of transmission from person to person. The virus is normally ingested from contaminated hands, food, milk, or water. Eating raw clams and oysters is also a risk factor for hepatitis A. HAV may also enter the body during sexual contact. Transmission from blood transfusion is rare. After an incubation period of 14 to 30 days, the virus invades hepatocytes (liver cells) causing inflammation and sometimes tissue death (necrosis). Virus is shed in the stool from 1–2 weeks to 5–6 weeks post-infection. Few patients die from hepatitis A. The hepatocytes eventually regenerate with little or no permanent damage, and patients who recover from the disease exhibit lifelong immunity to reinfection. Hepatitis A is much more contagious than hepatitis B, although less severe.

SIGNS AND SYMPTOMS: Malaise, anorexia, nausea, abdominal discomfort, and fever appear abruptly, followed in a few days by clay-colored stools and dark urine. Although jaundice is frequently apparent in the skin and sclera of the eye, it is not an indicator of the severity of the disease. The liver becomes enlarged and tender, and the spleen may also be enlarged. The contagious phase of hepatitis A usually lasts from three to six weeks. The convalescent phase may last 2 to 12 weeks, and recovery is usually complete.

LABORATORY DIAGNOSIS: ELISA tests are available which detect IgM or IgG antibodies to the hepatitis A virus. IgM is present in the serum from about 1 month to 5 months post-infection. Detection of IgM is diagnostic of a current or recurrent infection and detection of IgG indicates a previous hepatitis A infection.

PREVENTION AND TREATMENT: Education about good sanitation and personal hygiene, especially the proper disposal of bodily wastes, is the most effective means of prevention. Chlorination of drinking water inactivates hepatitis A virus. Injections of pooled human immunoglobulin (immune serum globulin) may prevent hepatitis A for up to six months. Since there is no specific treatment for hepatitis A, supportive care and bed rest are recommended.

Hepatitis B Gk. *hepatos*, liver; *itis*, inflammation

DEFINITION: Inflammation of the liver caused by the *hepatitis B virus* (HBV); also known as *serum hepatitis*.

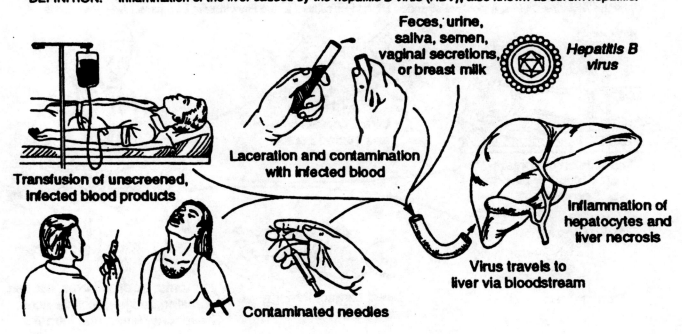

Feces, urine, saliva, semen, vaginal secretions, or breast milk

Hepatitis B virus

Transfusion of unscreened, infected blood products

Laceration and contamination with infected blood

Contaminated needles

Virus travels to liver via bloodstream

Inflammation of hepatocytes and liver necrosis

DESCRIPTION: The HBV is a double-stranded DNA *hepadnavirus* with a 27 nm nucleocapsid core surrounded by a complex lipoprotein coat. The entire 42 nm particle is known as a *Dane particle*. Transmission of the HBV is almost exclusively parenteral, meaning that the virus must breach the skin. Routes of infection include transfusion of blood and blood products, contaminated needles, coitus, and contamination of abrasions or lacerations with infected blood. Homosexuals, hemophiliacs, and health care workers are considered at high risk for contracting hepatitis B. Following an incubation period of 50 to 180 days, the virus invades hepatocytes (liver cells), causing inflammation and tissue death (necrosis). Hepatitis B is a more severe illness than hepatitis A, and some cases progress rapidly to death due to acute necrosis of the liver. Some patients may recover but remain in a persistent carrier state. Cirrhosis and hepatocellular carcinoma are secondary disorders which may result from HBV infection.

SIGNS AND SYMPTOMS: The onset of hepatitis B is insidious (the patient is unaware of infection) with malaise, anorexia, nausea, headache, and abdominal discomfort. The symptoms are replaced in a few days by clay-colored stools, dark urine, jaundice, and an enlarged and tender liver. Severity varies widely.

LABORATORY DIAGNOSIS: ELISA tests are available that detect the major HBV antigenic markers and antibodies to them. HBsAg is produced in the infected liver and spills into the blood, hence, screening blood for HBsAg detects most cases of acute and chronic hepatitis B; and detects most units of contaminated blood. The presence of anti-HBs shows recovery from HBV infection, or vaccination. Presence of HBeAg indicates active replication; anti-HBe indicates early recovery and a good prognosis. Anti-HBc is present during the acute phase and early recovery.

PREVENTION AND TREATMENT: Precautions should be taken to prevent transmission from contaminated needles or other equipment which might pierce the skin. Sharing needles among drug users must also be prevented, and blood bank products should be screened to eliminate blood contaminated with HBsAg. Hepatitis B component and recombinant vaccines are available. Healthcare and laboratory workers should be vaccinated. Although treatment is mainly supportive, hepatitis B immunoglobulin can be useful in therapy.

Hepatitis C (Non A–Non B Hepatitis) Gk. *hepatos*, liver; *itis*, inflammation

DEFINITION: An inflammation of the liver that is the most common post transfusion hepatitis in the U.S.; caused by the *hepatitis C virus*, a positive-stranded RNA virus related to the flaviviruses; also called *NANB hepatitis*.

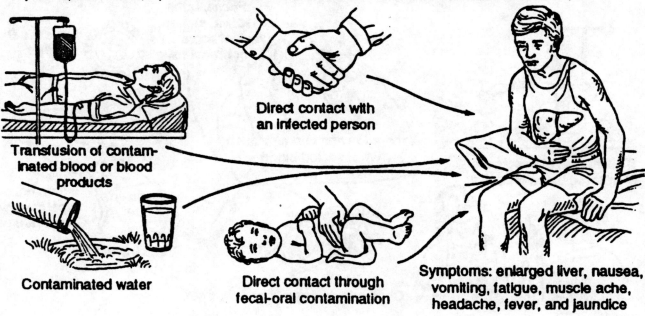

Transfusion of contaminated blood or blood products

Direct contact with an infected person

Contaminated water

Direct contact through fecal-oral contamination

Symptoms: enlarged liver, nausea, vomiting, fatigue, muscle ache, headache, fever, and jaundice

---

DESCRIPTION: Hepatitis C accounts for 90% of the cases of post transfusion hepatitis in the U.S. It is also spread by contaminated water, person to person contact, and by the fecal-oral routes. Hepatitis is usually a mild disease, but may be particularly severe when it occurs in the third trimester of pregnancy. Fatality rate may reach 10% in these cases. Epidemics of hepatitis C-like agents are common in India and South Asia. This condition clinically resembles hepatitis B, however there are no specific clinical features that distinguish hepatitis C from type A or B.

SIGNS AND SYMPTOMS: Hepatitis C may occur at any age and is characterized by a slow onset, anorexia, nausea, vomiting, fatigue, malaise, muscle and joint pain, headache, and photophobia. Later in the course of the disease, clay colored stools and dark urine are present. Systemic signs include fever, jaundice, and an enlarged liver. Complications include cirrhosis and hepatocellular carcinoma.

LABORATORY DIAGNOSIS: Diagnosis is made by eliminating the diagnoses of hepatitis A and hepatitis B; and obtaining a positive test for hepatitis C. The test for hepatitis C is an ELISA test that detects antibodies to hepatitis C virus.

PREVENTION AND TREATMENT: The disease is usually self limited. Preventative techniques include educating the public against multiple uses of hypodermic syringes and needles. Careful blood screening, especially high risk commercial blood, should be routinely carried out. There is no specific treatment for acute viral hepatitis so symptoms must be treated symptomatically.

Histoplasmosis Gk. *histos*, tissue; L. *plasma*, form; Gk. *osis*, condition

DEFINITION: A systemic respiratory disease caused by the dimorphic fungus *Histoplasma capsulatum*. This respiratory infection is worldwide in its occurrence and is common in birds and mammals, including man.

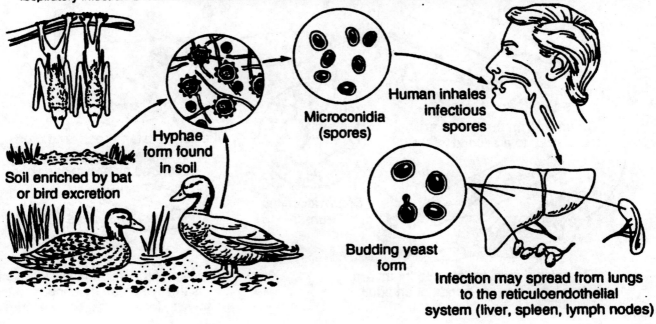

Soil enriched by bat or bird excretion

Hyphae form found in soil

Microconidia (spores)

Human inhales infectious spores

Budding yeast form

Infection may spread from lungs to the reticuloendothelial system (liver, spleen, lymph nodes)

DESCRIPTION: Histoplasmosis is a widely distributed, commonly occurring mycosis. The causative agent, *H. capsulatum*, is abundant in most soils that are enriched by the droppings of bats or birds. The organism develops in hyphal form and produces infectious conidial spores. When inhaled, the reticuloendothelial system is infected. In the lung the fungus develops as a budding, oval yeast. This fungus always exists as a yeast within the body of its host and as a mold in nature. Person to person transmission does not occur. In endemic areas, 80% of the adults have positive tests for this fungus infection and effective cellular mediated immunity is essential in controlling the fungal invasion. Histoplasmosis exists in primary, reinfection, chronic, disseminated, and ocular forms. In primary cases, an immune response induces delayed hypersensitivity to histoplasmin, which is an antigen derived from cells of the fungus. Disseminated disease indicates an underlying cell-mediated immune deficiency.

SIGNS AND SYMPTOMS: Most infections (at least 90%) are mild or asymptomatic. When symptoms do occur, they can vary from mild and self-limited to severe and fatal. Fever, anemia, and enlargement of the spleen and liver are evident in the severe form of the disease. Leukopenia, adrenal necrosis, pulmonary involvement (including multifocal cavitation and calcification), and ulcers of the GI tract are also possible.

LABORATORY DIAGNOSIS: Diagnosis depends on demonstrating or culturing *H. capsulatum* from involved tissues. The histoplasmic skin test is seldom useful because positive results are common in endemic areas. Serological tests are of some value.

PREVENTION AND TREATMENT: Soil contaminated with bird and bat droppings should be avoided such as roosting sites, chicken coops with old accumulations of droppings, and bat infested caves. Masks should be worn if these areas are unavoidable. Therapy is not usually indicated in mild primary histoplasmosis. Amphotericin B given intravenously can be helpful in the progressive disease. Surgical removal of the diseased tissue may become necessary. There is no vaccination available.

Impetigo L. *impeto*, a scabby eruption

DEFINITION: A highly contagious bacterial skin infection caused by staphylococci and streptococci. Impetigo is most common in newborns and children, and it resembles crusted brown sugar.

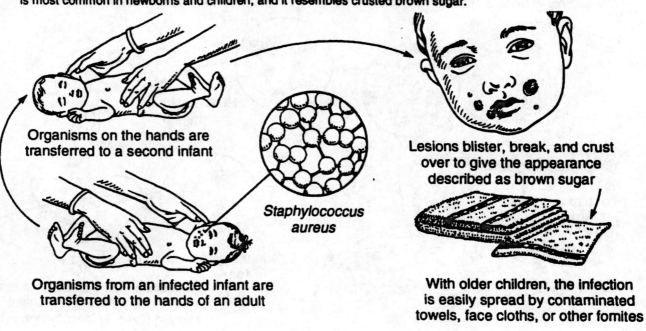

Organisms on the hands are transferred to a second infant

Organisms from an infected infant are transferred to the hands of an adult

Staphylococcus aureus

Lesions blister, break, and crust over to give the appearance described as brown sugar

With older children, the infection is easily spread by contaminated towels, face cloths, or other fomites

DESCRIPTION: Humans are the principal host of impetigo. Although occurring worldwide, this bacterial infection is mainly a problem in schools, camps, hospitals, and nurseries. The rash is rarely serious, but is highly contagious and can spread rapidly from one child to another. The bacteria are spread mainly by the hands and are rarely airborne. Lesions are most commonly found in diaper areas and the umbilical region in smaller children though they may be distributed anywhere on the body. Older children usually have lesions around the lips, nose, and ears.

SIGNS AND SYMPTOMS: Impetigo begins as a rash of small blisters that break and crust over to become yellow-brown scabs that look like brown sugar. The blistered area is surrounded by a puffy red base. Rupture of the pustules may cause peripheral spread of the condition, and is the period when the disease is most contagious. Complications are unusual, although pneumonia, septicemia, meningitis, and brain abscesses have been reported.

LABORATORY DIAGNOSIS: Diagnosis is made by bacteriologic culture, which may show either group A streptococci or *Staphylococcus aureus*. It is generally believed that streptococcus is the primary pathogen. Antibiotic sensitivity testing of the isolate determines the antibiotic of choice for treatment.

PREVENTION AND CONTROL: In a hospital nursery, the caregivers should wash their hands carefully before contact with each infant. "Rooming in" of infants with their mothers keeps the infants separate and decreases the possible spread of the infection. If impetigo is suspected, children should be kept home from school until they see a doctor. The rash can be treated by carefully removing crusts and cleaning skin well. The infected area should then be treated with an antibiotic ointment 3–4 times a day. Disseminated lesions usually respond well to systemic antibiotic (e.g. penicillin) therapy.

Infectious Mononucleosis Gk. *monos*, single: *nucleus*, kernel

DEFINITION: An acute, disseminated infectious disease caused by the *Epstein-Barr virus* (EBV), a herpes-group virus. It has also been designated the *kissing disease* because it is spread by mouth to mouth contact; also called *mononucleosis* or "*mono.*"

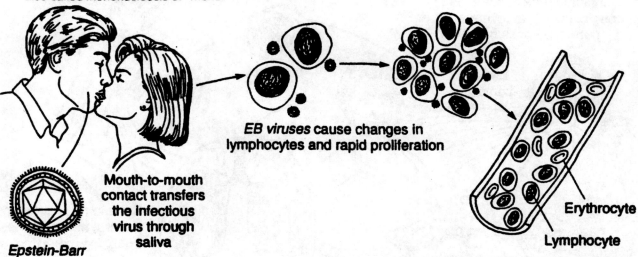

EB viruses cause changes in lymphocytes and rapid proliferation

Mouth-to-mouth contact transfers the infectious virus through saliva

Epstein-Barr

Erythrocyte

Lymphocyte

Greater ratio of lymphocytes in circulatory system brings about abnormal liver function

DESCRIPTION: This disease usually affects children and young adults (< 30 years old), with the highest incidence in the age range of 15 years to 25 years among higher socioeconomic groups. In developing nations, infection commonly occurs early in life and is largely asymptomatic. The virus is found in the oropharynx, lymphoid tissue and saliva of an infected person and is spread through saliva. However, it is not considered very contagious. EBV in the blood changes lymphocytes into rapidly proliferating cells causing an abnormally high number of mononuclear leukocytes in the blood. Abnormal liver function can occur in 90% of cases.

SIGNS AND SYMPTOMS: Fatigue, lack of energy, and malaise are the initial symptoms. A mild fever, sore throat, enlarged spleen and lymph nodes are also characteristic signs. The symptoms usually clear up in two to three weeks, sometimes longer. Recurrent episodes occur as latent viruses reactivate. Fatigue may be evident during recurrence.

LABORATORY DIAGNOSIS: The most common diagnostic features of the disease are the presence of certain heterophile antibodies in the blood and the presence of atypical lymphocytes. The heterophile antibodies are not virus-specific, but are induced in the majority of EBV infections. Tests such as the *monospot test* detect heterophile antibody. Diagnosis is also made using immunofluorescence tests which detect IgM and IgG antibodies to the EBV antigens; viral capsid antigen (VCA), EBV early antigen (EA), and EBV nuclear antigen (EBNA).

PREVENTION AND TREATMENT: There is no specific therapy for this condition. Bed rest and analgesics for sore throat pain help with the symptoms. Young children seem to recover more quickly. Recovery does confer immunity to mononucleosis. No vaccine is currently available. If serious complications develop (for example, hemolytic anemia, pharyngeal swelling interfering with swallowing), then cortisone is indicated. Humans are the only host for this disease.

Influenza Italian *influenza*, influence

DEFINITION: A highly communicable viral infection of the respiratory tract that has a seasonal occurrence during the winter months. It is caused by influenza viruses, members of the *orthomyxovirus* family.

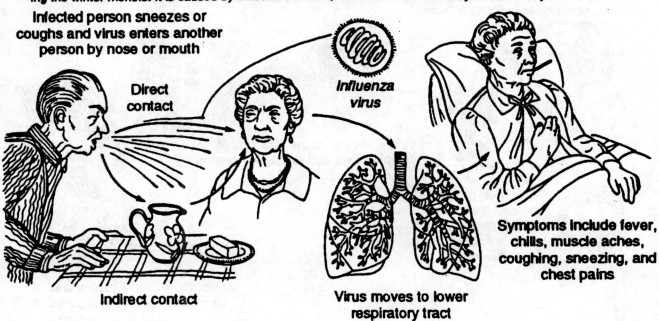

Infected person sneezes or coughs and virus enters another person by nose or mouth

Direct contact

Influenza virus

Indirect contact

Virus moves to lower respiratory tract

Symptoms include fever, chills, muscle aches, coughing, sneezing, and chest pains

DESCRIPTION: Influenza outbreaks usually occur in the fall and winter months. Every few years there is a major epidemic outbreak, or pandemic. The pandemic that occurred in the years 1918–1919 is the most famous appearance of influenza. During this time 200 million cases were reported and 50 million deaths occurred. It is highly contagious and spreads by direct and indirect contact. Influenza viruses enter by the mouth and nose and spread when an infected patient sneezes or coughs. Cigarette smoking increases the susceptibility to infection. Influenza viruses also tend to mutate readily. The virus contains a segmented single-stranded RNA genome containing 10 genes on 8 RNA segments. There are three major antigenic markers: the internal antigen, the external hemagglutinin (H), and neuraminidase (N) glycoprotein spikes. The three influenza types (A,B, and C) are based on differences in the internal antigen. Other subtypes are based on antigenic polymorphisms in H and N which are manifestations of the antigenic changes that occur because of antigenic drift (mutations) and antigenic shift (recombinations).

SIGNS AND SYMPTOMS: Influenza begins with a sudden onset of fever, chills, and muscle aches. It may be accompanied by pharyngitis or gastrointestinal upset. A 3–5 day period of illness is common, recovery is slow, and relapses may occur. The lower respiratory tract becomes involved if the airway is inflamed, causing coughing and continuous chest pain. Mortality is high in the elderly and those with cardiopulmonary disease. Influenza pneumonia or secondary bacterial pneumonia are possible serious complications.

LABORATORY DIAGNOSIS: Diagnosis is made by isolation of influenza virus in cell culture, demonstration of virus antigens in nasopharyngeal cells by immunofluorescence, or by demonstrating an antibody rise in paired sera.

PREVENTION AND TREATMENT: Avoiding contact with an infected person is the best means of prevention. After an attack, the patient acquires immunity against the same or closely related strains. New virus strains appear frequently, however, which may infect immune persons. When an epidemic strikes, prophylactic immunization with the appropriate H and N types will usually help to check it. Symptomatic care including bedrest and fluid replacement are important. The antiviral agent symmetrel is of some value in elderly patients. Aspirin should not be used as it is associated with development of Reye's syndrome in children.

Kuru (meaning shiver or tremble in the Fore language)

DEFINITION: A degenerative, fatal neurological disease which affects only members of the primitive Fore tribe inhabiting the remote eastern highlands of Papua, New Guinea.

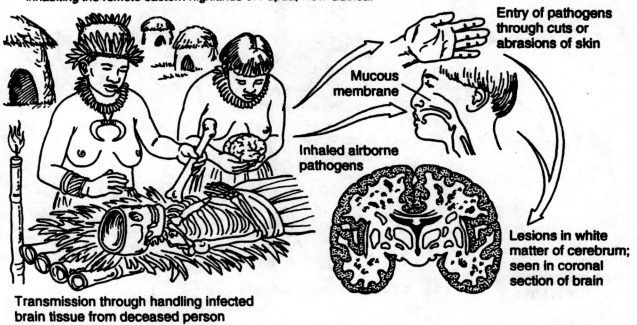

Entry of pathogens through cuts or abrasions of skin

Mucous membrane

Inhaled airborne pathogens

Lesions in white matter of cerebrum; seen in coronal section of brain

Transmission through handling infected brain tissue from deceased person

DESCRIPTION: During the late 1950's and early 1960's Kuru was the leading cause of death in the Fore tribe of New Guinea, affecting mainly young children of both sexes and adult women at an annual death rate of 2–3%. Ritual cannibalism, regularly practiced as a rite of mourning in the tribe until recently, is thought to be the route of transmission of the disease. Women and children were the major participants in those ceremonies, and their extensive handling of infected brain tissues, including smearing them upon the body, provided opportunity for the Kuru agent to enter the body through breaks in the skin and mucous membranes. Consumption of infected tissues appeared not to be a major factor in transmission of the disease. No one in contact with the living victims ever contracted Kuru, and the incidence of the disease diminished as cannibalism declined. These facts are evidence that transmission is limited exclusively to cannibalistic rites. The infectious agent for Kuru has yet to be isolated or visualized. It has been classified as a *slow virus* or *unconventional virus* or *prion* because of its unique properties, including resistance to inactivation, small size, and incubation period of 4 to 30 years. Kuru attacks the central nervous system (CNS) and causes a general loss of neurons, yet no inflammation is observed, and the cerebrospinal fluid remains normal. The cerebral hemispheres usually appear normal also, while the cerebellum is atrophied. *Status spongiosus*, in which the gray matter takes on an uncharacteristic spongy appearance, is common.

SIGNS AND SYMPTOMS: The early stages of Kuru are recognized by clumsiness and the inability to maintain balance. Loss of muscle coordination, changes in mood and personality, and slurred speech follow. The disease progresses rapidly and is characterized by fine shivering tremors. Death normally occurs 3 to 9 months after the onset of symptoms.

LABORATORY DIAGNOSIS: No routine diagnostic tests are available.

PREVENTION AND TREATMENT: Prevention is possible by departure from traditional treatment of the dead within the Fore tribe. No effective treatment for Kuru is known.

Lassa Fever (from Lassa, Nigeria where disease was first described)

DEFINITION: A hemorrhagic fever most common in West Africa; caused by a rodent-borne *arenavirus*.

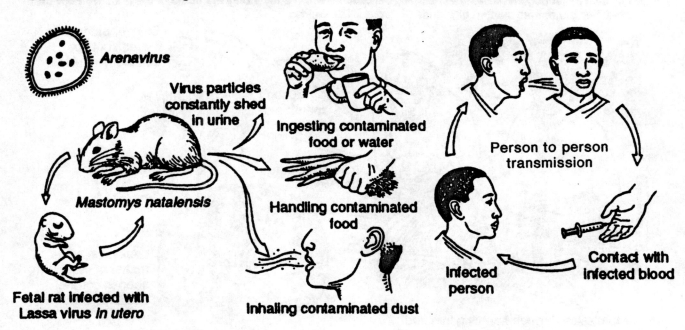

Arenavirus

Virus particles constantly shed in urine

Ingesting contaminated food or water

Handling contaminated food

Person to person transmission

Mastomys natalensis

Fetal rat infected with Lassa virus *in utero*

Inhaling contaminated dust

Infected person

Contact with infected blood

DESCRIPTION: Lassa fever is caused by a single-stranded RNA pleomorphic *arenavirus*, 80–150 nm in diameter. The rodent *Mastomys natalensis* is the natural reservoir for this causative agent. The rodents acquire a chronic infection *in utero*, and virus particles are shed in their urine throughout life. Humans contract the virus through cuts in the skin while handling food contaminated with rodent urine, ingesting contaminated food or water, or by inhaling contaminated dust. In addition, the rat-like rodents are a major food item for many people in West Africa. When the route of infection is the upper respiratory system or ingestion, the primary site of viral infection is the oropharynx. Following an incubation of 3 to 16 days, the virus extends into the circulatory system causing systemic infection. Person to person transmission through contact with infected blood, excretions, or respiratory droplets is the factor that distinguishes Lassa virus from other arenaviruses.

SIGNS AND SYMPTOMS: Fever, muscle and joint pain, and diarrhea are early symptoms of both mild and serious illness. Serious cases accelerate toward the end of the first week with severe sore throat, chest and abdominal pain, and vomiting. Signs of subcutaneous bleeding known as *petechiae* may sometimes be seen in the skin of the face, neck, shoulders, and back. Widespread internal bleeding can also occur, and death due to shock and cardiovascular collapse occurs in 30 to 50% of these cases. Vertigo and tinnitus may appear during the second or third week of milder illness, and these cases can result in permanent deafness. The overall mortality rate for victims of Lassa fever is less than 5%.

LABORATORY DIAGNOSIS: Diagnosis can be made by detecting anti-viral IgM or IgG in immunofluorescence tests, or by isolating Lassa fever virus in cell culture from blood, cerebrospinal fluid, or throat washings.

PREVENTION AND TREATMENT: Controlling rodent populations, avoiding consumption of *M. natalensis* as a food source, and protecting food stores from contamination are the best preventive measures. Transmission from person to person is prevented by isolating infected patients and requiring barrier precautions—gowns, gloves, and masks—for all persons who come in contact with patients or their laboratory specimens. The drug ribavirin is an effective treatment for Lassa fever, generating a 5 to 10% decrease in fatality.

Legionellosis

DEFINITION: An acute bacterial pneumonia that was first discovered in a group attending the July 1976 convention of the American Legion in Philadelphia. It is caused by the gram negative bacilli *Legionella pneumophila, L. bozemanii, L. micdadei;* and other species of *Legionella;* also called *Legionnaires' disease.*

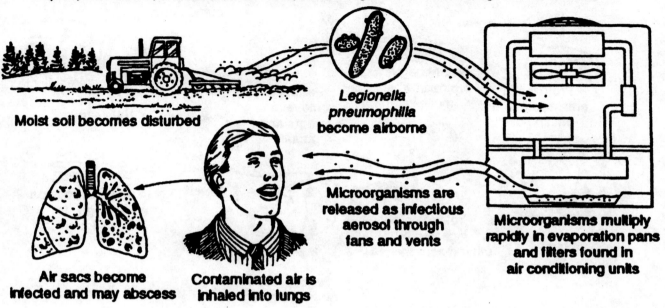

Moist soil becomes disturbed

Legionella pneumophilla become airborne

Microorganisms multiply rapidly in evaporation pans and filters found in air conditioning units

Microorganisms are released as infectious aerosol through fans and vents

Air sacs become infected and may abscess

Contaminated air is inhaled into lungs

DESCRIPTION: The bacilli that cause legionellosis have been recovered from water in air conditioning cooling units. The bacilli grow initially in the moist soil and become airborne when soil is disturbed. They then spread into evaporation pans and filters of large air conditioning units where they multiply rapidly in the correct temperature and humidity. Later, the organisms are released in an infectious aerosol through fans and exhaust vents of the system. Inhalation of contaminated air is the mode for acquiring the infectious agents. Legionellosis is not spread from an infected person to a non-infected person. The air sacs in both lungs of patients fill with an exudate composed of neutrophils, macrophages, and fibrin. Sometimes abscesses may form. There are an increased number of cases of legionellosis during summer months, and this disease was probably the one implicated in unsolved epidemics going back to 1965.

SIGNS AND SYMPTOMS: The condition begins with malaise, muscle aches, and a slight headache. A day after onset, a rapidly rising temperature and shaking chills appear. A non-productive cough then leads to a productive cough. Pneumonia develops within a week. Mortality is 15% with death due to respiratory failure or shock.

LABORATORY DIAGNOSIS: Specific diagnosis is made by isolation of *Legionella* from respiratory secretions, lung tissue, pleural fluid, or blood; detection of specific antigens in appropriate specimens, or demonstration of a significant rise in antibody titer during convalescence.

PREVENTION AND TREATMENT: Cooling systems of large buildings and hospitals should be periodically checked for the presence of *L. pneumophila.* If present, the system should be disinfected. Actual incidence of legionellosis is low. Convalescent patients develop antibodies against the infectious organism. Erythromycin is the antibiotic of choice but rifampin can also be used effectively.

Leishmaniasis after William B. Leishman, British physician, 1865–1926

DEFINITION: An infection with a species from the genus *Leishmania*, which are parasitic flagellate protozoa. The condition occurs in subtropical and tropical climates and is transmitted by the bite of the female sandfly of the genus *Phlebotomus*.

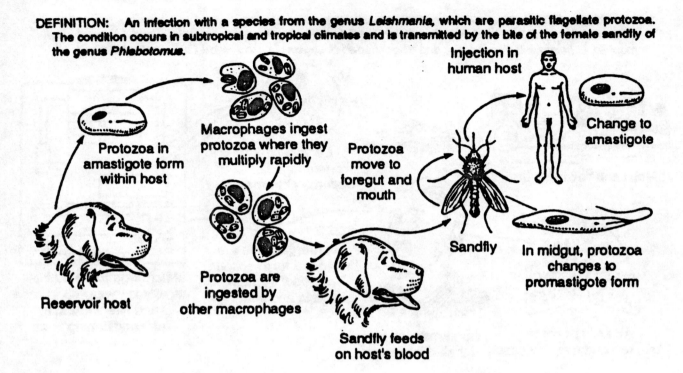

DESCRIPTION: There are two types of leishmaniasis: *cutaneous* and *visceral*. The cutaneous form frequently causes disfiguring ulcers. The visceral form afflicts internal body organs and is the more serious of the two. Dogs and rodents are also affected with this disease and are frequently the reservoir host as the infection is transmitted through the bite of a sandfly vector. The protozoa exist in the vertebrate host in the amastigote form. Here they are ingested by macrophages where they multiply rapidly. After the infected macrophages die, the protozoa are ingested by other macrophages. When the female sandfly feeds on blood, the protozoa move into the insect's midgut. Here they emerge from the macrophages, transform into promastigote forms by elongating and developing a flagellum, and continue to multiply. Eventually the protozoa move forward through the insect's gut to the foregut and mouth, from which they can be injected through the sandfly's next victim. In the patient, the organism changes into the amastigote form again. Transmission may also occur if the fly's body is crushed on the skin during feeding. Blood transfusion from an infected host is also a mode of disease transmission.

SIGNS AND SYMPTOMS: Lesions develop around the bite of the vector. They can heal spontaneously, or the healing can be followed by a latent period and then by eruption of ulcers on the mucous membranes of the nose, mouth, respiratory tract, or vagina. If the disease remains untreated, extensive tissue destruction, disfigurement, and death may occur. The cutaneous form exhibits nodular and ulcerating lesions in the skin and mucous membranes. The visceral type of the disease is characterized by fever, enlargement of the spleen and liver, progressive emaciation, weakness, and eventually death. Mortality may be as high as 75% to 90% in untreated patients of visceral leishmaniasis.

LABORATORY DIAGNOSIS: A positive leishmanin skin test and serum antibody indicates current or previous infection. Impression smears may contain amastigotes, but culture is the most sensitive method.

PREVENTION AND TREATMENT: Avoiding areas where the vector lives and avoiding contact with the sandfly vector are the main methods of prevention. Stibogluconate sodium is the CDC drug of choice. Pentostam and other antimalarial drugs have also been used.

Leprosy (lep'ro-se) Gk. *lepros*, scaly

DEFINITION: A slowly progressive, communicable infection manifested in two principal forms: tuberculoid and lepromatous; caused by the acid-fast bacillus *Mycobacterium leprae*; also known as *Hansen's disease.*

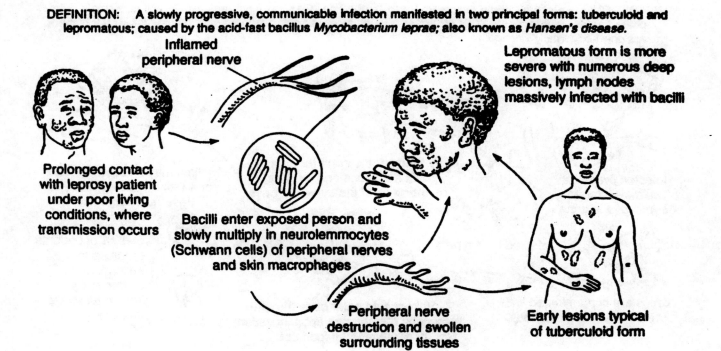

Inflamed peripheral nerve

Prolonged contact with leprosy patient under poor living conditions, where transmission occurs

Bacilli enter exposed person and slowly multiply in neurolemmocytes (Schwann cells) of peripheral nerves and skin macrophages

Peripheral nerve destruction and swollen surrounding tissues

Lepromatous form is more severe with numerous deep lesions, lymph nodes massively infected with bacilli

Early lesions typical of tuberculoid form

DESCRIPTION: Leprosy has been feared for more than 25 centuries. The bacilli present in the lesions of the skin and in mucous membranes are spread by person to person contact, however, the exact means of transmission is unknown. The incubation period is very long and highly variable. Once the bacilli enter the body they multiply in neurolemmocytes (Schwann cells) at peripheral nerve endings and cause nerve destruction. Tissue supplied by the nerves becomes swollen, enlarged, insensitive and may be inadvertently damaged. Much of the tissue damage is due to secondary invasion by other opportunistic microorganisms. The *tuberculoid (neural) form* of leprosy is milder, characterized by skin depigmentation and loss of sensation. The *lepromatous (progressive) form* is usually disseminated since disfiguring nodules form all over the body. Patients with the lepromatous form have diminished cell-mediated immune responsiveness and the disease has progressed from the tuberculoid stage.

SIGNS AND SYMPTOMS: The signs and symptoms of this disease have a gradual onset. Tumor-like growths appear on the skin and mucous membranes. Localized areas of skin anesthesia are present. Untreated patients are characterized by extreme deformity and destruction of tissue.

LABORATORY DIAGNOSIS: Acid-fast bacilli may be detected by the Ziehl-Neelsen stain in smears of nasal scrapings and the buffy coat of blood. Skin biopsies are also examined for bacilli.

PREVENTION AND TREATMENT: Good living conditions are important, and prolonged and intimate contact with leprosy patients is hazardous, although leprosy is not as contagious as once believed. Once the disease has been contracted, dapsone and rifampin are the anti-bacterial drugs of choice. Children living with leprous parents should be medicated prophylactically. With proper therapy the disease can often be controlled. Except for the armadillo, humans are the only host of leprosy. Because of this, armadillos are frequently used to test medications and vaccines.

Leptospirosis Gk. *leptos*, slender; *speira*, coil; *osis*, condition

DEFINITION: An acute, febrile disease caused by the fine (0.15 μm diameter), tightly coiled, aerobic spirochete *Leptospira interrogans*. This organism is found in wild and domestic animals all over the world; humans are only accidentally infected.

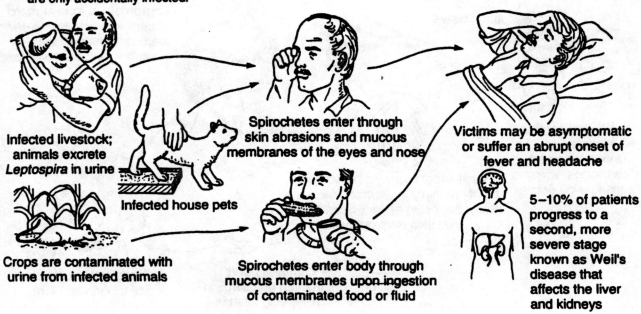

Infected livestock; animals excrete *Leptospira* in urine

Infected house pets

Crops are contaminated with urine from infected animals

Spirochetes enter through skin abrasions and mucous membranes of the eyes and nose

Spirochetes enter body through mucous membranes upon ingestion of contaminated food or fluid

Victims may be asymptomatic or suffer an abrupt onset of fever and headache

5–10% of patients progress to a second, more severe stage known as Weil's disease that affects the liver and kidneys

DESCRIPTION: *Leptospira interrogans* are contained in the urine of infected animals and are usually transmitted to other hosts via this medium. Humans may acquire leptospirosis by contact with infected animals, their urine, or soil infected with contaminated urine. The organism enters the host through a surface abrasion or through the mucous membranes of the eyes, nose, and mouth. No lesion appears at the point of organism entry. In severe cases, the basement membranes in the kidneys may be destroyed causing a decreased filtering ability, a condition called *Weil's disease*.

SYMPTOMS: Leptospirosis is generally a monophasic illness, but in a few patients it is characterized by two stages. Abrupt onset of fever and severe headache typify the first stage. Muscular pains, redness of the conjunctiva, myalgia, jaundice, tenderness and either diarrhea or constipation may also occur. Aseptic meningitis is a possible complication. The second stage begins after a brief afebrile period. At this time the microorganisms are developing and multiplying in the renal tubules. The fever then returns, followed by meningitis, hepatomegaly, and hepatic tenderness. These are the symptoms of the advanced and more severe stage of leptospirosis, called Weil's disease. Approximately 5–10% of all cases of leptospirosis advance to this stage.

LABORATORY DIAGNOSIS: Diagnosis may be confirmed by culture (on Fletcher's semisolid medium) or blood or urine. Serological tests detecting IgM antibody or a rise in total antibody titer are diagnostic. Direct examination of urine for the leptospires is not sufficient to establish the diagnosis.

PREVENTION AND TREATMENT: To prevent leptospirosis, avoid rat infested areas and swimming in contaminated water. Incidence of this disease is highest in the summer and fall months. Survival of an attack of leptospirosis promotes lasting immunity. Occupations at risk include sewer workers, farmers, and veterinarians. Penicillin, doxycycline, and tetracycline are the treatments of choice and must be given early in the course of the disease. Dialysis is a supportive measure that has been effective in severe cases. Vaccines are available for the immunization of animals.

Lyme Disease

DEFINITION: A tick-borne disease caused by the spirochete *Borrelia burgdorferi.* Lyme disease was first recognized in the U.S. in 1975 in a group of children in Lyme, Connecticut.

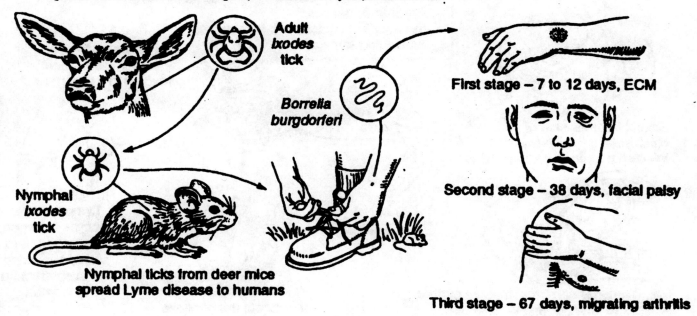

Adult Ixodes tick

Borrelia burgdorferi

Nymphal Ixodes tick

Nymphal ticks from deer mice spread Lyme disease to humans

First stage – 7 to 12 days, ECM

Second stage – 38 days, facial palsy

Third stage – 67 days, migrating arthritis

DESCRIPTION: *Borrelia burgdorferi* is transmitted mainly through the ticks *Ixodes dammini* (Northeast and upper Midwest) and *Ixodes pacificus* (Northern California coast). The adult ticks feed on deer, but it is the nymphal, comma-sized ticks which feed on deer mice, *Peromyscus maniculatus*, that are usually responsible for spreading the disease to humans. The bite of the tick is usually painless, and they can feed from their host in less than one hour. Lyme disease is endemic not only in the U.S., but also in parts of Europe and Asia.

SIGNS AND SYMPTOMS: Lyme disease is described in three stages:
First stage—a "bull's-eye" rash, or erythema chronicum migrans (ECM), that appears within days to weeks—or not at all—around a papule at the site of the tick bite. This stage is also characterized by fever, headaches, malaise, dizziness, and stiff neck.
Second stage—B. burgdorferi enters the CNS which may result in neurologic and cardiac disorders such as facial palsy and heart arrhythmias.
Third stage—swollen and painful joints that may develop into migrating arthritis.

LABORATORY DIAGNOSIS: Diagnosis is made by detecting specific IgM or IgG antibodies in the serum. ELISA tests or immunofluorescence tests are commonly used. Culture for the spirochetes is rarely successful.

PREVENTION AND TREATMENT: The best method of prevention is to avoid being bitten by ticks when camping or hiking in endemic areas. Wearing protective clothing and using arthropod repellents is advisable. It is also important to inspect clothing and the entire body surface for the presence of ticks following campouts or picnics in locations known to be infected with ticks. Lyme disease is usually treated with high doses of phenoxymethyl penicillin or tetracycline. Penicillin G is used in stage 2 and stage 3 infections.

Lymphogranuloma Venereum L. *lympha*, lymph; *granulum*, grain; *oma*, tumor

DEFINITION: Lymphogranuloma venereum (LGV) is a subset of the most common sexually transmitted disease, the *chlamydial infections,* which may result in male or female infertility.

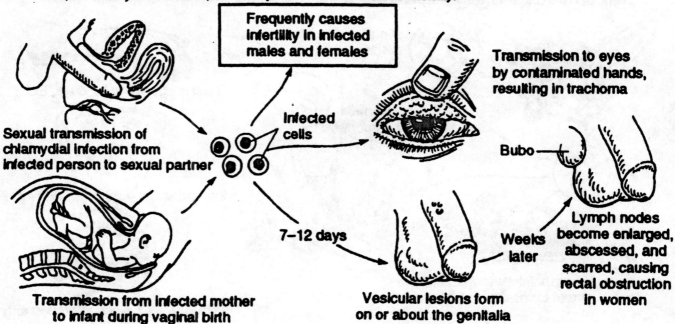

Frequently causes infertility in infected males and females

Sexual transmission of chlamydial infection from infected person to sexual partner

Transmission from infected mother to infant during vaginal birth

Infected cells

7–12 days

Vesicular lesions form on or about the genitalia

Transmission to eyes by contaminated hands, resulting in trachoma

Bubo

Weeks later

Lymph nodes become enlarged, abscessed, and scarred, causing rectal obstruction in women

DESCRIPTION: The chlamydiae are nonmotile, gram-negative, obligate intracellular bacteria. They cannot synthesize their own ATP and are, in a sense, energy parasites. They replicate within the cytoplasm of host cells, forming characteristic inclusions. The family *Chlamydiaidae* consists of the genus *Chlamydia,* and three species, *C. trachomatis, C. psittaci,* and *C. pneumoniae.* Included within the species *C. trachomatis,* are the organisms causing trachoma (chronic follicular conjuctivitis—the most common preventable worldwide cause of blindness), inclusion conjunctivitis, LGV (serotypes L1, L2, and L3), and other genital tract chlamydia. LGV and the other genital tract chlamydia are distributed worldwide, and humans are the only known carriers. They are spread through sexual intercourse but can also be transmitted during birth to the baby. LGV infections are also common in homosexual males. Patients with *Chlamydia* frequently have other sexually transmitted diseases concurrently, especially syphilis and gonorrhea.

SIGNS AND SYMPTOMS: From 7–12 days after exposure, a person with LGV experiences fever, headaches, and myalgia. About this time, a small, vesicular lesion appears on or about the genitals. This ruptures and heals painlessly. Then from one to eight weeks later, the genital and inguinal lymph nodes enlarge, become tender, and may suppurate. At this stage, the enlarged lymph nodes are called buboes. Buboes may also develop into abscesses and form draining fistulas. When buboes heal they leave scars that may obstruct lymph channels. The perirectal lymph nodes in women may scar and cause rectal obstruction. The non-LGV strains are less severe and may manifest simply as urethritis, cervicitis, or may be inapparent. Epididymitis and acute salpingitis may also occur causing reproductive sterility.

LABORATORY DIAGNOSIS: Diagnosis is best accomplished by culture tests performed in cell culture. Direct smears, antigen-detecting EIA's, and nucleic acid probes are also used. Serological tests detecting anti-LGV antibodies give useful information.

PREVENTION AND TREATMENT: The best prevention is to know one's sexual partner and to use condoms which protect somewhat against the spread of sexually transmitted diseases. Tetracyclines and sulfonamide drugs are effective against LGV. Untreated LGV may relapse and become chronically active, capable of infecting a sexual partner many years after the initial infection.

Malaria L. *malum*, an evil; *aria*, air

DEFINITION: An infectious disease of humans and other animals caused by *Plasmodium* protozoa. Transmission occurs as an infected *Anopheles* mosquito injects sporozoites into the bloodstream of a person; also called *blackwater fever*, or *jungle fever*.

Oocysts form from zygote; sporozoites develop in oocyst, which ruptures to release sporozoites in salivary glands of mosquito

Sporozoites infect hepatocytes and produce merozoites by asexual fission; some merozoites infect other hepatocytes and others penetrate erythrocytes

Sporozoite

Oocyst

Zygote

Mosquito biting

Fertilization

Gametes

Hepatocyte (liver cell)

Merozoite

Liver

Erythrocyte

Mosquito bites infected person and sucks up blood with gametocytes; gametes form and are fertilized to become zygote in mosquito's digestive tract

Mosquito biting

Gametocyte

Merozoites rapidly increase in numbers through asexual reproduction as they feed on hemoglobin; merozoites also infect other erythrocytes, which rupture releasing merozoites

DESCRIPTION: Human malaria is caused by four species of *Plasmodium*: *P. vivax*, *P. malariae*, *P. ovale*, and *P. falciparum*. Infections from *P. falciparum* account for about 50% of the malaria cases and are the most life-threatening. When an infected *Anopheles* mosquito bites a victim, she injects saliva containing anticoagulant and haploid *sporozoites*. Once in the human bloodstream, the sporozoites are transported to the hepatocytes (liver cells) where they undergo asexual fission (*schizogony*) and produce *merozoites*. The merozoites then infect other hepatocytes or penetrate erythrocytes. Once within an erythrocyte, a merozoite becomes an ameoboid *trophozoite*, feeding on hemoglobin. The nucleus of a trophozoite then divides, producing a multinucleated *schizont*. Further divisions produce mononucleated merozoites. Eventually, the erythrocyte ruptures releasing merozoites, toxins, and cell debris. Some of the merozoites do not rupture erythrocytes, but rather differentiate into *macrogametocytes* and *microgametocytes*. If an *Anopheles* mosquito feeds on a malaria victim, the macrogametocytes and microgametocytes will develop into female and male gametes, respectively, within the mosquito. A diploid zygote, called an *ookinete*, forms in the mosquito's gut. An oocyst develops from the ookinete and eventually ruptures releasing sporozoites, some of which penetrate the mosquito's salivary glands.

SIGNS AND SYMPTOMS: The signs and symptoms of malaria include the sensation of intense cold and shivering, followed by a rapid rise in temperature to 104° to 106° F. This is followed by an intense headache with mild delirium. There are typically 48 hours between attacks. Death is usually due to cardiovascular problems, including the loss of erythrocytes.

LABORATORY DIAGNOSIS: Diagnosis is made from identification of malarial parasites on a Giemsa-stained thick and thin blood film.

PREVENTION AND TREATMENT: An estimated 100 million people are infected with malaria, and over one million of these die annually. Controlling mosquito populations through spraying and draining of swamps, and the avoidance of mosquito infested areas, are somewhat effective in prevention of malaria. Antimalarial drugs such as *chloroquine*, *amodiaquine*, and *primaquine* are frequently used, but there are many plasmodium strains that are resistant to each, or several, or all, of these drugs.

DEFINITION: An acute, highly communicable disease most common in school-aged children. It is caused by the *rubeola virus* (a *paramyxovirus*); also called *rubeola*.

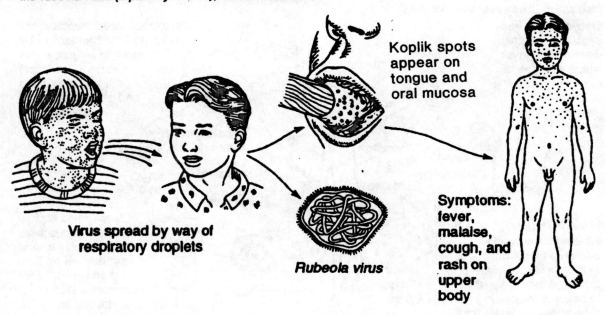

Koplik spots appear on tongue and oral mucosa

Virus spread by way of respiratory droplets

Rubeola virus

Symptoms: fever, malaise, cough, and rash on upper body

DESCRIPTION: The measles virus is found in respiratory tract secretions, blood, and urine. It is usually transmitted by contact with an infected patient through respiratory droplets. Once it enters a host, the incubation period is 10–12 days. The virus begins to multiply in the respiratory mucosa while the disease is still asymptomatic. It then spreads via the bloodstream to the skin and other areas of the body through a *viremic stage* where the characteristic red spots are expressed. The virus multiplies most effectively in epithelial and neural tissues. Measles is more severe in infants and adults than in children. Measles outbreaks are most common in the winter and early spring, and are worldwide in occurrence.

SIGNS AND SYMPTOMS: Measles begins with fever, malaise, cough, and conjunctivitis. Small, irregular bluish-red spots, called *Koplik spots*, are present on the buccal mucosa. This is followed by the eruption of a rash that begins on the face and spreads onto the torso and appendages. The rash lasts from 4–5 days, does not itch, and as it subsides the body temperature also declines. Photophobia is a prominent characteristic of this infection. Encephalitis, pneumonia, and otitis media are possible complications of measles. Mortality in the U.S. is less than 1%, but may reach 10% in developing countries.

LABORATORY DIAGNOSIS: Diagnosis is made by detecting anti-viral IgM antibodies in serum or detecting a rise in IgG antibody titer in paired sera. Isolation of virus from the nasopharynx or from blood is possible but frequently unsuccessful.

PREVENTION AND TREATMENT: All children should be immunized for measles with a live virus vaccine (commonly included in the mumps-measles-rubella, or MMR vaccine) given at 12 months to 15 months of age. Treatment of measles includes bed rest and antipyretics given to treat directly the symptoms. Antibiotics may also be given to prevent secondary bacterial infection which can be common in children. Measles infection almost invariably confers life-long immunity.

Meningitis (men-in-ji'tis) Gk. *meninx*, membrane; *itis*, inflammation

DEFINITION: An inflammation of the membranes of the spinal cord or brain. It can be caused by bacteria, viruses or other organisms that reach the meninges via blood, lymph, or fractured bone.

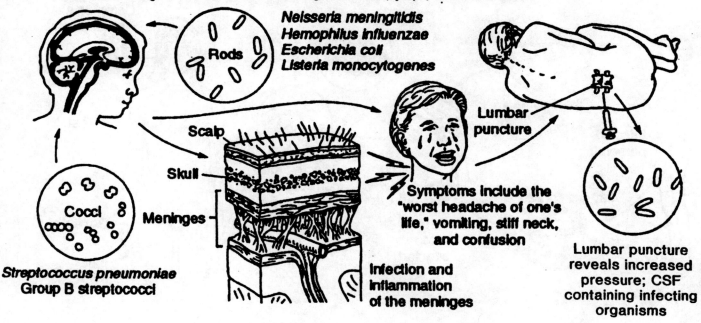

Neisseria meningitidis
Hemophilus influenzae
Escherichia coli
Listeria monocytogenes

Rods

Scalp

Skull

Meninges

Cocci

Streptococcus pneumoniae
Group B streptococci

Symptoms include the "worst headache of one's life," vomiting, stiff neck, and confusion

Infection and inflammation of the meninges

Lumbar puncture

Lumbar puncture reveals increased pressure; CSF containing infecting organisms

DEFINITION: There are three main types of infections that cause meningitis. *Bacterial infections* are one type with *Neisseria meningitidis* (the meningococci) and *Hemophilus influenzae* being the causes of the epidemic form of meningitis. The *tubercle bacillus* causes the second type of meningitis infection, and the third types are *viral*, or *aseptic*. In infants other bacteria, such as streptococci and gram-negative bacilli, are etiologic agents. Meningitis is primarily a childhood condition with 90 percent of all cases occurring between the ages of one month to 5 years. The organisms usually reach the meninges due to the secondary spread of infections or through trauma.

SIGNS AND SYMPTOMS: The diagnostic symptoms are due to the increased intracranial pressure caused by the inflammation of the meninges. These symptoms include moderate and irregular fever, loss of appetite, and intense headache. Intolerance to light and sound and nuchal rigidity are also common. Pupils may be contracted, and with extreme infections, convulsions and even coma may be evident.

LABORATORY DIAGNOSIS: A lumbar puncture is necessary to correctly diagnose the illness, during which cerebrospinal fluid (CSF) pressure and presence of the infecting organism are noted. Bacteria may be found in stained smears on cultured or laboratory media. An elevated leucocyte level and a low glucose level in the CSF indicate a bacterial etiology.

PREVENTION AND TREATMENT: The HIB vaccine has been developed to protect children from bacterial meningitis caused by *Hemophilus influenzae* Type B. Recently, the *H. influenzae* type B conjugate vaccine (HbCV) has been developed. All children between 2 months and 5 years of age should be vaccinated. Meningitis requires early recognition and immediate therapy to prevent death and to avoid residual disabilities. Antibiotics such as ampicillin, penicillin G, and gentamicin are used if the organism is susceptible. Supportive symptomatic therapy is also indicated to reduce the intracranial pressure and to treat headache pain. Patients with this condition should be isolated.

Molluscum Contagiosum (mo-lus'kum) L. *molluscum*, soft

DEFINITION: A mildly contagious skin disease that affects mainly children and young adults; caused by a large virus of the pox group. It is characterized by small, waxy, globular epithelial tumors.

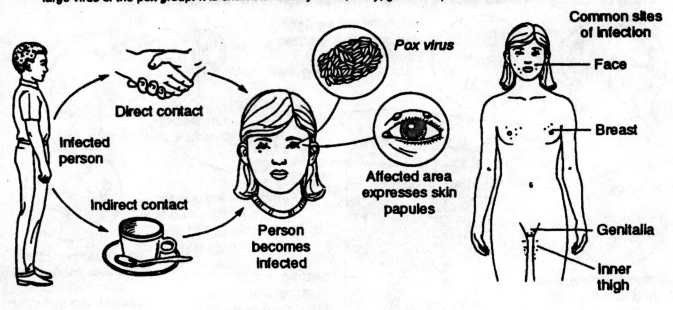

DESCRIPTION: This condition is spread from person to person by direct and indirect contact. It is an uncommon viral infection characterized by the occurrence in children of one or more small, dome-shaped skin tumors. It occasionally develops in scratched areas of patients with atopic eczema.

SIGNS AND SYMPTOMS: The waxy, translucent, skin colored raised papules vary in diameter from 2 mm to 5 mm. They are rarely larger. The lesions contain semifluid caseous matter or solid masses. They heal without scarring though they may suppurate and break down. Common areas for the infection to occur are the face, eyelids, breasts, genitalia, and inner surfaces of the thigh. The infected areas may become inflamed from secondary bacterial infection.

LABORATORY DIAGNOSIS: Molluscum contagiosum can be diagnosed easily by the characteristic central umbilication of the papule, filled with a semisolid white material that, if expressed and Giemsa-stained, shows many large cells containing inclusion bodies.

PREVENTION AND TREATMENT: Prevention is through avoidance of direct contact with a patient during the infectious stage of the disease. Treatment includes incision of the lesions and expression of the contents, followed by the application of tincture of iodine. Electrosurgery can also be done lightly and rapidly—only enough to induce trauma to the lesion. Trauma can cause the lesion to disappear. They must not be completely destroyed by electrosurgery, as is the treatment for warts.

Mumps Eng. *mump*, a lump or bump

DEFINITION: An acute, contagious, febrile disease characterized by painful, inflammatory swelling of one or both parotid salivary glands; caused by the mumps virus (a *paramyxovirus*); also called *epidemic parotitis*.

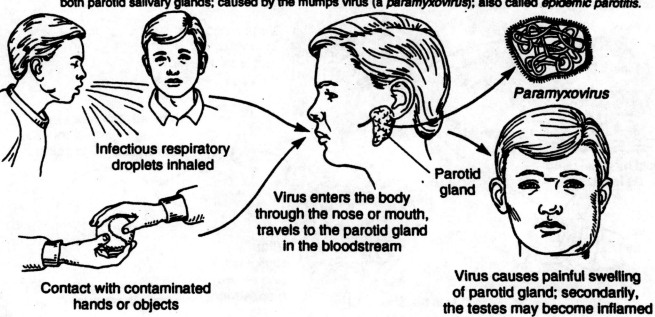

Infectious respiratory droplets inhaled

Contact with contaminated hands or objects

Virus enters the body through the nose or mouth, travels to the parotid gland in the bloodstream

Paramyxovirus

Parotid gland

Virus causes painful swelling of parotid gland; secondarily, the testes may become inflamed

DESCRIPTION: Mumps usually occurs in children between the ages of 5 and 15 years. When adult epidemics occur, they are extremely difficult to control. The mumps virus is transmitted from person to person directly by drops of saliva and indirectly from contaminated hands and objects. The virus enters the body through the mouth and reaches the parotid gland through the bloodstream. Here it multiplies and causes extreme inflammation and swelling. Infections of the submaxillary and sublingual glands are also possible but not as common. Mumps may be unilateral or bilateral, affecting one or both sides of the face.

SIGNS AND SYMPTOMS: The symptoms begin gradually with chilliness, malaise, headache, pain below the ears, and moderate fever. This is followed by swelling of one or both parotid glands and jaw movements become very painful and restricted. Swelling lasts from 5–7 days. After puberty, a serious complication for male patients is orchitis, or inflammation of the testes, which may lead to sterility. Mumps encephalitis may also rarely occur.

LABORATORY DIAGNOSIS: Clinical diagnoses of mumps can be confirmed in the laboratory by isolation of mumps virus in cell culture from saliva, materials collected from around the parotid (Stensen's) duct of the parotid gland, cerebrospinal fluid, or urine. Serological diagnosis can be made by demonstrating a significant rise in antibody titer between acute and convalescent sera.

PREVENTION AND TREATMENT: Because mumps is an infectious disease, isolation of a patient with mumps during the infectious stage will control its spread. A highly effective live virus vaccine is available, the mumps-measles-rubella (MMR) vaccine, and is recommended for all children and others who may be susceptible, especially males. Bed rest, a soft diet and analgesics for pain are important to control symptoms of mumps. Cold local applications may also control swelling of salivary glands. Life-long immunity follows recovery from the disease. Mothers with immunity also confer six months of protection to their infants.

Myocarditis Gk. *myo*, muscle; *kardia*, heart; *itis*, inflammation

DEFINITION: An inflammation of the myocardium of the heart that is associated with a number of conditions including many types of infections.

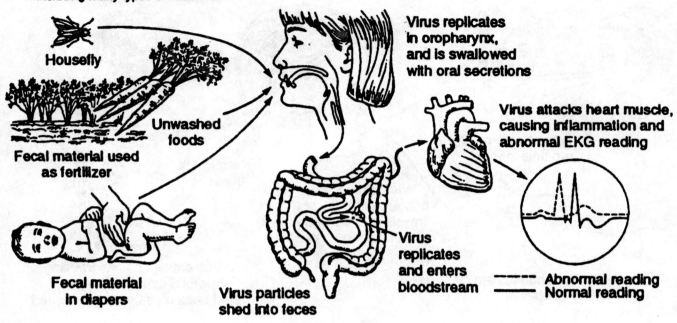

Housefly

Unwashed foods

Fecal material used as fertilizer

Fecal material in diapers

Virus particles shed into feces

Virus replicates and enters bloodstream

Virus replicates in oropharynx, and is swallowed with oral secretions

Virus attacks heart muscle, causing inflammation and abnormal EKG reading

- - - - Abnormal reading
———— Normal reading

DESCRIPTION: The term *myocarditis* is a complicating secondary infection to primary conditions elsewhere in the body. A patient afflicted with myocarditis has a reduced contractility of the heart. Nephritis, infections, carbon monoxide poisoning, heat stroke, and burns are some conditions that may lead to myocarditis. Myocarditis occurs commonly after rheumatic fever and diphtheria. The tertiary stage of syphilis can also lead to this problem. In the U.S. and Western Europe, infectious myocarditis is most commonly due to enterovirus infection, especially the Group B coxsackie viruses. Group A coxsackie viruses and echoviruses are involved to a lesser extent. Some manifestation of myocarditis may also be idiopathic.

SIGNS AND SYMPTOMS: A patient with myocarditis has a weak and rapid heart beat, especially at the apex of the heart. The pulse is also irregular and weak. There is extreme tenderness over the precordium, or area of the chest above the heart. The patient manifests dyspnea and fatigues very easily. General malaise also accompanies the condition. The patient with myocarditis may recover spontaneously, may recover but never have normal heart function, or may die from the disease.

LABORATORY DIAGNOSIS: Diagnosis of microbial etiologies of myocarditis is often difficult as culture testing is frequently negative because myocarditis may occur long after initial infection. Cultures for enteroviruses may provide positive results when the myocardium, the pericardium, or pericardial fluid is cultured. Isolation of virus from throat or stool along with rises in titer of anti-viral antibodies provides circumstantial evidence.

PREVENTION AND TREATMENT: The main method of prevention is to avoid or treat quickly the causative problems. Rheumatic fever and diphtheria should especially be avoided by use of vaccines (DPT for diphtheria) and general sanitation. Syphilis should be treated in its early stages. Treatment of myocarditis consists of bedrest in order to minimize cardiac work load. Antibiotics may be administered if the cause is bacterial. Corticosteroids are also given to decrease the inflammatory process. Patients with myocarditis should be monitored for life-threatening dysrhythmias so that they can be treated immediately.

Otitis Media Gk. *otos*, ear; *itis*, inflammation; *media*, middle

DEFINITION: Common inflammation of the middle ear caused by a variety of organisms including *Streptococcus pneumoniae, Haemophilus influenzae, Streptococcus pyogenes*, and *Staphylococcus aureus.*

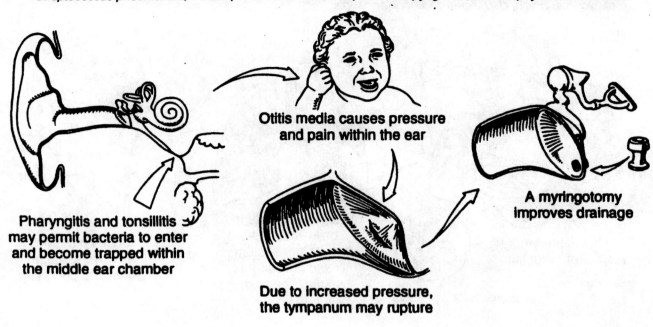

Pharyngitis and tonsillitis may permit bacteria to enter and become trapped within the middle ear chamber

Otitis media causes pressure and pain within the ear

Due to increased pressure, the tympanum may rupture

A myringotomy improves drainage

DESCRIPTION: Otitis media often develops from pharyngitis or tonsillitis. Swelling of the tonsils can block auditory (eustachian) tubes which contributes to entrapment of the infecting organisms in the middle ear. This condition affects small children almost exclusively due to the anatomical shape of their auditory tubes. Boys are affected more than girls and the incidence increases in the winter months. It is not uncommon for a child to have an ear infection more than once a year.

SIGNS AND SYMPTOMS: Signs and symptoms are pain in the ear, reddening and bulging of the tympanum (eardrum), and increased temperature. Fluid accumulates in the enclosed middle ear chamber. Infants who cannot communicate pain tend to hold or pull their ears and roll their head from side to side. The inflammation can cause perforation of the tympanum to relieve pressure and scarring may occur. Repeated or prolonged cases may lead to hearing loss. Meningitis and mastoiditis are possible complications.

LABORATORY DIAGNOSIS: Spontaneous otorrhea and the exudate obtained at myringotomy should be cultured. Nasopharyngeal cultures may be helpful but often do not correlate well with the causative organism.

PREVENTION AND TREATMENT: In many cases where the causative organism is unknown, a broad-spectrum antimicrobial agent, such as ampicillin, is prescribed. Recurrent or chronic cases are treated surgically by the installation of tympanotomy tubes in a procedure called a *myringotomy* to provide continual middle ear drainage. Warm application to the outer ear can relieve the pain. A vaccine is available for children to receive at two months of age that provides immunity to *H. Influenzae* (HbCV). It is recommended for all children. A pneumococcal vaccine is also available for high risk individuals.

Pertussis (per-tus′is) L. *per*, through; *tussis*, cough

DEFINITION: An acute respiratory infection which occurs chiefly in children under 4 years of age who have not been immunized; caused by *Bordetella pertussis*. It is highly contagious and characterized by a peculiar paroxysmal cough; also known as *whooping cough*.

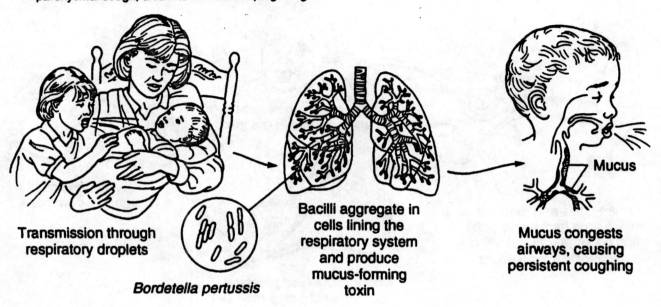

Transmission through
respiratory droplets

Bordetella pertussis

Bacilli aggregate in
cells lining the
respiratory system
and produce
mucus-forming
toxin

Mucus

Mucus congests
airways, causing
persistent coughing

DESCRIPTION: Pertussis is transmitted by airborne droplets from the upper respiratory tract and by objects recently contaminated with the bacterium *Bordetella pertussis*. *B. pertussis* is a small, gram-negative, non-motile, aerobic, rod. In the respiratory system, the bacilli accumulate in large masses among the cells lining the walls of the trachea and bronchi, where the bacteria produce toxins (both endotoxin and an exotoxin) which cause a thick, sticky mucus that congests the airways, causing the patient to go into the characteristic coughing episodes. This disease occurs worldwide and is particularly threatening to young infants.

SIGNS AND SYMPTOMS: The illness is typically divided into three stages. The *Catarrhal stage* exhibits signs and symptoms similar to the common cold such as increased fever, sneezing, irritability, dry cough and loss of appetite. The *Paroxysmal stage* sets in after about two weeks and consists of violent coughing spells. They begin with several short coughs, followed by a long drawn inspiration during which the typical whoop is heard. The number of paroxysms in 24 hours may vary from 3–4 up to 40–50. These coughing spells fail to expel the respiratory mucus and leave the patient exhausted. Cough is precipitated by eating, drinking and pressure on the trachea and it may be associated with vomiting. The Paroxysmal stage may endure for 1–2 months. The final stage is called the *Decline stage* when the paroxysms grow less frequent and less violent. Nutrition improves and then the cough finally ceases. Secondary complications may include bronchopneumonia and tuberculosis.

LABORATORY DIAGNOSIS: Culture of nasopharyngeal mucus on Bordet-Gengou medium or Regan-Lowe medium may grow *B. pertussis*. The organism is most easily recovered in the catarrhal or early paroxysmal stages.

PREVENTION AND TREATMENT: Newborns are very susceptible to pertussis and should therefore be isolated from an infected child. Erythromycin, tetracycline, or chloramphenicol can stop the growth of the *B. pertussis* but will not shorten the illness. A single episode of the disease confers life-long immunity. There is an effective vaccine available (Diphtheria-Pertussis-Tetanus, DPT). This vaccine should be administered to all infants four times starting at two months of age.

Plague L. *plaga*, a stroke

DEFINITION: A highly fatal infectious disease caused by the gram-negative coccobacillus *Yersinia pestis*. This intracellular parasite is transmitted to humans by the bites of infected fleas. Three pandemics of the plague in European history killed over 125 million people; also called *bubonic plague*, or *black death*.

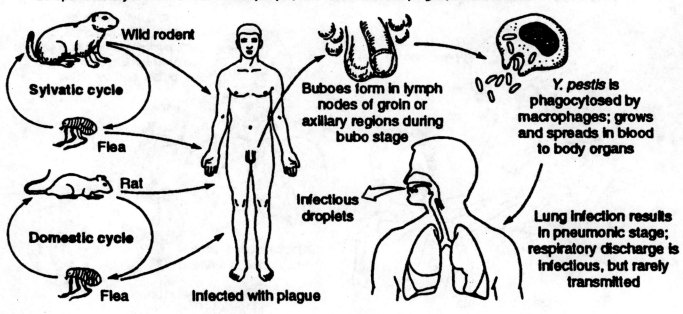

Wild rodent

Sylvatic cycle

Flea

Rat

Domestic cycle

Flea

Infected with plague

Buboes form in lymph nodes of groin or axillary regions during bubo stage

Infectious droplets

Y. pestis is phagocytosed by macrophages; grows and spreads in blood to body organs

Lung infection results in pneumonic stage; respiratory discharge is infectious, but rarely transmitted

DESCRIPTION: Plague was responsible for the deaths of millions of people during the Middle Ages; nearly one-fourth the population of Europe. Fleas on the fur of *Rattus norvegicus* were the principal vectors on the common rat host. There are three forms of plague, *bubonic, septicemic,* and *pneumonic*. In bubonic plague, bacteria invade regional lymph nodes causing them to become infected and swollen (the buboes). In septicemic plague, the bacteria are found in the blood. In pneumonic plague, the bacteria are concentrated in the lungs, having arrived there through inhalation of infectious respiratory droplets. Humans can contract plague from the bite of infected fleas. *Y. pestis* survives in fleas and rodents in either the *domestic cycle* or the *sylvatic cycle* (within wild populations), and can survive for long periods of time in hibernating hosts and in the soil of animal burrows. It is harbored in wild populations of rodents in the Southwest part of the U.S., particularly in ground squirrels, gophers, prairie dogs, chipmunks, and field mice.

SIGNS AND SYMPTOMS: The onset of plague is usually very sudden with chills, high fever, and malaise being the early signs and symptoms. This is followed by the *bubo stage* characterized by swollen and tender lymph nodes. Unless the buboes rupture, bubonic plague is likely not transmitted. Septicemic and pneumonic forms are highly infectious. Death occurs from the endotoxin and exotoxin produced by large populations of bacteria which leads to circulatory collapse and heart failure, or when septic emboli from buboes enter the respiratory system causing respiratory failure.

LABORATORY DIAGNOSIS: Diagnosis is made by culture isolation of bipolar staining short rods from buboes, aspirates, blood, or sputum. Fluorescent antibody staining confirms the identity of the isolate. Seroconversion is demonstrated by testing paired sera by the passive hemagglutination test.

PREVENTION AND TREATMENT: Since plague is transmitted by wild rodents and domestic rats, the disease can be prevented by avoiding dead, and possibly infected, rodents and by living in sanitary environments which preclude rats and fleas. The mortality rate for untreated bubonic plague is about 80%, and near 100% for untreated septicemic and pneumonic plague. If treated with streptomycin or tetracycline the mortality rate drops to near 20% in all cases. A vaccine has not been developed for long-term immunization, but vaccines are available for limited protection. There are fewer than 50 cases of plague yearly in the U.S.

Pneumonia (nu-mo′ne-a) Gk. *pneumon*, lung

DEFINITION: Inflammation of the lungs caused primarily by bacteria, viruses, protozoans, or chemical irritants. There are over 50 causes of pneumonia, however, 60–80% of cases are caused by the bacterium *Streptococcus pneumoniae*, a gram-positive, encapsulated *diplococcus*.

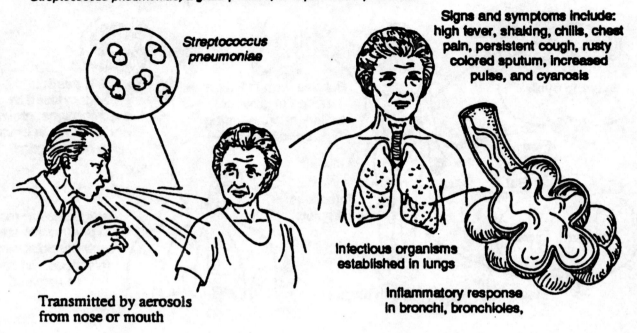

Streptococcus pneumoniae

Signs and symptoms include: high fever, shaking, chills, chest pain, persistent cough, rusty colored sputum, increased pulse, and cyanosis

Transmitted by aerosols from nose or mouth

Infectious organisms established in lungs

Inflammatory response in bronchi, bronchioles,

DESCRIPTION: Infectious agents causing pneumonia are transmitted by aerosols from the nose or mouth and in sputum. Organisms of the normal flora may cause pneumonia in immunocompromised patients. When the microorganism establishes itself in the lungs, it causes an inflammatory response in the bronchi, bronchioles, and alveoli of the lungs. These structures then become congested with a fibrinous exudate. Leukocytes and macrophages aggregate to destroy the pathogens but add to the problem by enhancing tissue destruction as they release proteolytic enzymes. Capsules surrounding *S. Pneumoniae* enhance bacterial virulence by protecting against phagocytosis. The microorganisms compete with lung cells for nutrients, decrease the available oxygen, and increase blood acidity. Complications of pneumonia include bacteremia which may lead to meningitis, endocarditis, pleurisy, or arthritis.

SIGNS AND SYMPTOMS: A shaking chill and high fever along with a pleuritic type of chest pain are the first symptoms of pneumonia. A productive cough is also present and may produce rusty colored sputum. The victim exhibits rapid, shallow breathing, an increased pulse, cyanosis, and an increased blood leukocyte count. Mortality is high if not treated with an appropriate antibiotic.

LABORATORY DIAGNOSIS: The most common bacterial pathogens causing pneumonia are *S. pneumoniae, H. influenzae, S. aureus, Legionella pneumophilia,* and *Mycoplasma pneumoniae.* Differential diagnosis is made by culture isolation of the pathogen from sputum or blood. Antibiotic sensitivity testing on the isolate should be performed to identify an effective antibiotic for therapy.

PREVENTION AND TREATMENT: Most healthy people have resistance to pneumonia. However, weak, malnourished, alcoholic, sick, and aged people are at risk for acquiring pneumonia and must be guarded while under medical care. A vaccine against *S. pneumoniae* is available for high risk patients. Penicillin, tetracyclines, cephalosporins, and erythromycin may be used for treatment, depending upon the microbial diagnosis. Antibiotics are not useful in treating viral pneumonia, except to prevent secondary bacterial invasion. Complete recovery with no residual lung damage is possible.

Poliomyelitis (pol"e-o-mi"el-i'tis) Gk. *polios*, gray; *myelos*, marrow

DEFINITION: An acute infectious disease caused by the *poliovirus* of the *picornavirus* group, that affects nervous tissue causing paralysis and permanent muscle atrophy or death; also called *polio*, or *infantile paralysis*.

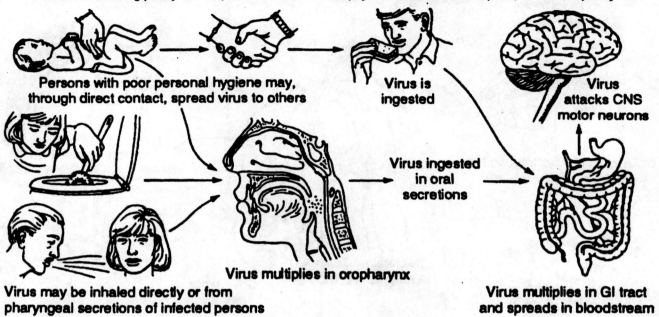

Persons with poor personal hygiene may, through direct contact, spread virus to others

Virus is ingested

Virus attacks CNS motor neurons

Virus ingested in oral secretions

Virus may be inhaled directly or from pharyngeal secretions of infected persons

Virus multiplies in oropharynx

Virus multiplies in GI tract and spreads in bloodstream

DESCRIPTION: The poliovirus is a type of *picornavirus* composed of a single-stranded RNA genome with an icosahedral capsid and a diameter of about 27 nm. There are three strains of the polio virus: *Type I* is highly contagious, but causes only moderate paralysis; *Type II* occurs sporadically, but causes the greatest numbers of paralytic victims; and *Type III* occurs sporadically, remains in the GI tract, rarely causing paralysis. The poliovirus gains entry into the GI tract through contaminated fluid or food. From here, the viruses multiply and may infect the tonsils and lymphatic tissues of the oropharynx and GI tract. Movement of the viruses through the bloodstream to nervous tissues leads to the more critical stage of the disease. Polioviruses multiply rapidly in motor neurons (the gray matter) of the medulla oblongata and spinal cord. It is estimated that a single virus may produce over 250,000 new virions during a single replication cycle. The most serious form of infection occurs in the medulla oblongata resulting in a condition called *bulbar polio* because of the bulblike appearance of the medulla. The disease is more severe in older patients than in infants because of maternal antibodies in babies. Poliomyelitis is spread by contaminated feces of carriers or the inhalation of respiratory droplets from an infected person.

SIGNS AND SYMPTOMS: Most cases of polio are asymptomatic and the afflicted person simply develops immunity. In many polio patients, the symptoms include GI tract discomfort and respiratory infection, but no central nervous system involvement. If the CNS is involved, loss of muscle function occurs and irreversible paralysis and deformity frequently result. Cases are fatal when vital autonomic functions in the brain are lost, such as control over respiratory movement. Only 1 in every 100 cases is paralytic.

LABORATORY DIAGNOSIS: Diagnosis is made by culture isolation of poliovirus from respiratory or stool specimens, or by detection of seroconversion or antibody rise in acute and convalescent sera.

PREVENTION AND TREATMENT: Recovery from disease gives life-long immunity. Two types of vaccines exist: inactivated polio vaccine (IPV, or *Salk vaccine*), and oral live-virus vaccine (OPV, or *Sabin vaccine*). Both of these vaccines are trivalent in that they confer immunity to the three types of poliovirus. OPV is the vaccine of choice in the U.S. All infants (except immunodeficient children) should receive the vaccine even though there is a slight risk that the attenuated virus can revert to its virulent form and cause disease. Unsanitary swimming areas and consumption of contaminated shellfish have been identified as risk factors for polio infection.

Psittacosis (sit-a-ko'sis) Gk. *psittakos*, parrot; *osis*, condition

DEFINITION: An influenza-like infectious disease caused by the bacterial organism *Chlamydia psittaci*. It primarily affects parrots and other birds, but it may be transmitted to humans; also called *ornithosis, chlamydiosis,* or *parrot fever.*

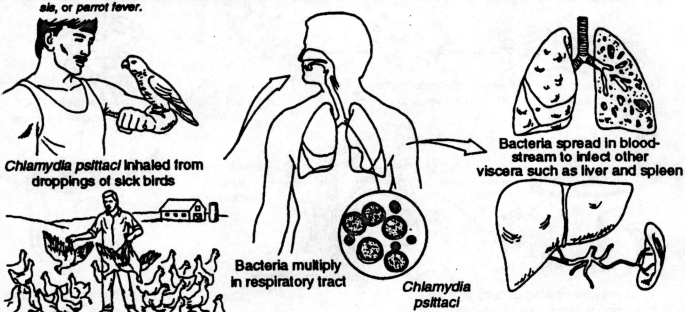

Chlamydia psittaci inhaled from droppings of sick birds

Bacteria multiply in respiratory tract

Chlamydia psittaci

Bacteria spread in bloodstream to infect other viscera such as liver and spleen

DESCRIPTION: The causative agent, *C. psittaci*, is an obligate intracellular bacterium. Transmission of psittacosis to humans may occur from handling sick birds and their feathers, by contact with materials that have been contaminated by birds, inhalation of dried bird excreta, and from bites or wounds inflicted by sick birds. The infected birds show *Chlamydia* in their nasal discharge and in their feces from an infected GI tract. Humans are infected through their respiratory tract where the organisms become localized. Transmission of psittacosis can occur from person to person. Psittacine birds, most often parrots and parakeets, are the principal carriers of the disease. *Ornithosis* is the name given to this disease in domestic fowl.

SIGNS AND SYMPTOMS: The signs and symptoms of psittacosis in humans include headache, epistaxis, nausea, chill followed by fever, constipation, and sometimes pulmonary disorders. The condition is characterized by a sudden onset and it can spread via the blood to involve other organs, particularly the liver and the spleen. A pneumonitis could occur accompanied by a severe cough. A high mortality rate exists if the infection is allowed to spread systemically.

LABORATORY DIAGNOSIS: Diagnosis is generally made by a four-fold rise in complement-fixing antibodies in paired sera. Culture isolation of *C. psittaci* is possible in cell culture, but should be attempted only in specialized laboratories.

PREVENTION AND TREATMENT: The safest prevention is simply to avoid contact with sick birds. People who must work in close contact with birds should take precautions to avoid the inhalation of dust from feces. Tetracyclines, erythromycin, and penicillin are the antibiotics of choice. No vaccine is available.

Puerperal Sepsis (pu-er'per-al) L. *puer*, child; *parere*, to bring forth

DEFINITION: A condition of septicemia or infection following childbirth. The causative organisms are usually *Streptococci* or *Clostridia*; also called *childbed fever* or *peurperal fever*.

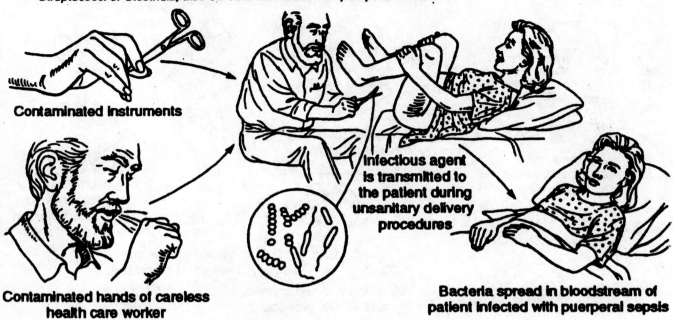

Contaminated instruments

Contaminated hands of careless health care worker

Infectious agent is transmitted to the patient during unsanitary delivery procedures

Bacteria spread in bloodstream of patient infected with puerperal sepsis

DESCRIPTION: In 1847, Ignaz Semmelweis, a Hungarian physician, demonstrated that acute puerperal sepsis was transmitted primarily by the hands of those attending women in labor. At this time, one of eight women having a hospital delivery died of septicemia. Currently, the occurrence of puerperal sepsis in hospital maternity wards is rare due to the current practice of asepsis and improved hygiene. Septicemia is common, however, with women who have illegal abortions, and frequently results in death. If a delivery or an abortion is performed in unsanitary conditions, an infection may start within 24–48 hours following the procedure. The causative organisms usually come from the nose and throat of the patient herself or from those attending her. *Streptococcus pyogenes* is a common causative organism. These pathogens reach the uterus through contaminated hands or instruments. The uterus is easily infected because it has been traumatized during the birth or abortion, and the separation of the placenta.

SIGNS AND SYMPTOMS: The signs and symptoms of puerperal sepsis include fever, leukocytosis, and pain and tenderness of the lower abdominal area and genital tract. The infection may spread through the cervical wall or through the uterine (fallopian) tubes, causing bacteremia or peritonitis. Death may occur unless antibiotic therapy is promptly instituted.

LABORATORY DIAGNOSIS: Vaginal exudates, lochia, and the urinary tract are cultured by aerobic and anaerobic culture. Isolated pathogens should be tested for antibiotic sensitivity in order to institute optimal therapy.

PREVENTION AND TREATMENT: Modern aseptic techniques used as a preventative measure could cause this condition to be nearly eliminated. Today, most postpartum infections are caused by *Escherichia coli* staphylococci, enterococci, anaerobic cocci, and *Bacteroides*. Prior to the development of antibiotics, streptococcal puerperal sepsis was almost inevitably fatal. Now, prompt therapy with penicillin or other appropriate antibiotics saves most patients with puerperal infection.

DEFINITION: An acute infectious disease caused by the rickettsial organism *Coxiella burnetii*. It infects a variety of animals, but unlike other rickettsial diseases it is not transmitted to humans through an insect vector.

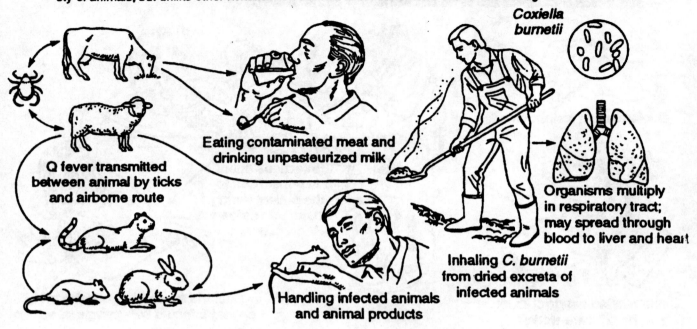

Coxiella burnetii

Q fever transmitted between animal by ticks and airborne route

Eating contaminated meat and drinking unpasteurized milk

Handling infected animals and animal products

Inhaling *C. burnetii* from dried excreta of infected animals

Organisms multiply in respiratory tract; may spread through blood to liver and heart

DESCRIPTION: Q fever usually infects domestic animals such as goats, cows, or sheep. Humans contract it by inhaling infected dust, drinking unpasteurized milk from infected animals, or by handling infected animals. Transmission from human contact is rare, but it has occurred. The disease is transmitted between animal hosts by infected ticks. Q fever is worldwide in distribution and is an atypical rickettsial disease because it is not transmitted to humans by insect vectors, and only rarely through tick vectors.

SIGNS AND SYMPTOMS: This disease is characterized by headache, fever, severe sweating, malaise, myalgia, and anorexia. The frontal headache may be accompanied by chills and pneumonia. Hepatitis and endocarditis may also result. Q fever has an abrupt onset and no rash occurs as with other rickettsial diseases. This febrile disease is self-limiting and of short duration.

LABORATORY DIAGNOSIS: Diagnosis is generally made using serology. A complement fixation test is available which detects antibodies to *C. burnetii* antigens.

PREVENTION AND TREATMENT: Since the *Coxiella burnetii* organisms are resistant to drying, infectious aerosols can be generated in handling of wool and from dried secretions and excreta from infected animals. An effective vaccine is available for persons who have a good chance of exposure to the disease. Infection is especially common among packing house employees and lab workers. Unpasteurized milk should also be avoided. Treatment of Q fever with the tetracyclines is effective.

Rabies L. *rabio*, to rage, fury

DEFINITION: A highly fatal infectious disease that may afflict all species of homeothermic (warm-blooded) animals, including man. It is caused by a neurotropic virus that occurs in the central nervous system (CNS) and is commonly transmitted in the saliva by the bite of a rabid animal; also called *hydrophobia*.

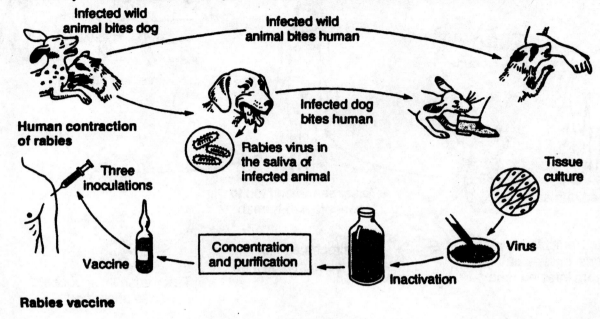

DESCRIPTION: Rabies is caused by the rabies virus, a *rhabdovirus*. It is bullet-shaped, contains a single-stranded RNA genome, and can be transmitted to humans through the saliva from the bite of an infected animal. Muscle and connective tissues at the wound site are initially infected and the disease remains localized for periods ranging from days to months. Eventually, the virus spreads via the bloodstream to the CNS where cytoplasmic inclusion bodies (*Negri bodies*) develop within the neurons of the brain and/or nerves. Once within the brain, the disease is considered fatal. In infected dogs, *furious rabies* implies aggressive and vicious behavior, while in *dumb rabies* paralytic symptoms predominate.

SIGNS AND SYMPTOMS: The incubation period for rabies is shorter in children than in adults. It also is dependent upon the location of the bite and the relative number of viruses transmitted through the wound. Clinical signs and symptoms include fever, headache, aggressive and irritable behavior, and sensitivity to light and sound. These symptoms are followed by *hydrophobia* (fear of water) because of difficulty in swallowing as pharyngeal muscles become paralyzed. Saliva drips from the mouth because it cannot be swallowed. As the disease progresses, there is general paralysis, coma, and death.

LABORATORY DIAGNOSIS: For diagnosis in animals, the brain tissue is examined by immunofluorescence for virus-infected cells, virus isolation is attempted, and tissue sections may be examined for the presence of Negri bodies. Diagnosis in humans is made by clinical evaluations and history of exposure. Post-mortem evaluation of brain tissue by culture and immunofluorescence may reveal the presence of rabies virus.

PREVENTION AND TREATMENT: Obvious prevention is the avoidance of wild animals that exhibit abnormal behavior and keeping pets away from contact with wild animals. Vaccination of pets against rabies is required in most cities. Because of the delayed spread of rabies to the brain following the bite of an infected animal, active immunization is used as a treatment after suspected infection (post-exposure immunization). The current rabies vaccine for human immunization (the *diploid vaccine*) is administered in 3 injections over a 7-day period.

DEFINITION: An infectious disease marked by intermittent attacks of high fever. It is caused by several species of the genus *Borrellia*, and it is transmitted by head lice, body lice, and ticks of the genus *Omithodoros*.

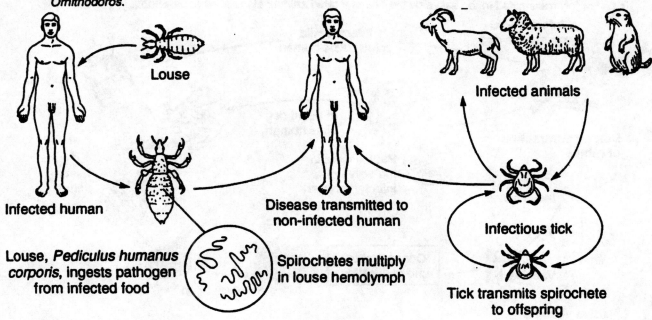

Louse

Infected animals

Infected human

Disease transmitted to non-infected human

Infectious tick

Louse, *Pediculus humanus corporis*, ingests pathogen from infected food

Spirochetes multiply in louse hemolymph

Tick transmits spirochete to offspring

DESCRIPTION: The *Borrellia* spirochetes are found in the blood of the mammalian host during fever and are transferred from person to person by body lice, *Pediculus humanus corporis*. After the organism is ingested by the louse, it travels to the insect's midgut where it penetrates the gut wall and enters the hemolymph where it multiplies rapidly. The louse will remain infected for life. When the lice are crushed on the skin, usually by scratching, the hemolymph is released and further hosts may become infected. Infected ticks may also transmit this disease from infected goats, sheep, and rodents such as ground squirrels, prairie dogs, and chipmunks. Ticks transfer the spirochetes through their saliva as they bite a host. Infected ticks may transmit the infection to their offspring for generation after generation. Lice do not transfer the infection to their offspring.

SIGNS AND SYMPTOMS: Relapsing fever is characterized by alternating periods of febrile illness with apparent recovery. The onset of fever is very sudden. This condition occurs most frequently in the summer months. Louseborne fever appears as an epidemic.

LABORATORY DIAGNOSIS: Diagnosis is made by demonstration of spirochetemia. This is done by preparing a thin film of peripheral blood, then staining it with Wright's stain or Giemsa stain, or by observing it by darkfield or phase contrast microscopy. The spirochetes are 5 to 20 μm in length and are observable lying in-between blood cells or overlying blood cells.

PREVENTION AND TREATMENT: Preventive measures include rodent control, the wearing of proper clothing, and the use of insecticides. Treatment of a patient with relapsing fever generally requires only a single dose of either tetracycline, erythromycin, or procaine penicillin G. Symptomatic treatment and supportive therapy is also helpful. The organisms are able to undergo antigenic variation within the host, so a successful vaccine has not been developed.

Respiratory Syncytial Disease Gk. *syn*, together; *kytos*, cell

DEFINITION: An acute lower respiratory disease of infants and children; caused by the *respiratory syncytial virus (RSV)* which is a *paramyxovirus*. Death from RSV may involve infection by other opportunistic organisms.

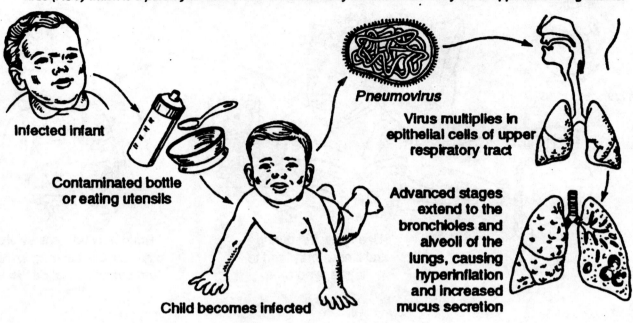

Infected infant

Contaminated bottle or eating utensils

Child becomes infected

Pneumovirus

Virus multiplies in epithelial cells of upper respiratory tract

Advanced stages extend to the bronchioles and alveoli of the lungs, causing hyperinflation and increased mucus secretion

DESCRIPTION: RSV belongs to the genus *Pneumovirus* in the family Paramyxoviridae. This disease is transmitted by close contact with an infected infant, child, or adult, or from fomites that have been contaminated by an ill person. Respiratory syncytial disease usually affects children before age four. Forty percent of RSV infections are nosocomial. The pathology accompanying this disease resembles an upper respiratory tract infection or a common cold, then may progress as the bronchi, bronchioles, and alveoli within the lungs become infected. Symptoms for adults are similar to a common cold. Viral replication is confined to the epithelial cells of the respiratory tract. The infected cells exhibit ballooning of their cytoplasm and syncytia may be observed as cell fusion occurs. The pathologic problems are caused as cells are shed into the lumina as they die, trapping air and causing hyperinflation and increased mucus secretion.

SIGNS AND SYMPTOMS: A variety of disease patterns may be caused by RSV including bronchiolitis and pneumonia. Symptoms for patients under three weeks of age include lethargy, irritability, and respiratory distress. Symptoms for patients older than three weeks of age include crackles, retractions, and manifestations of upper respiratory tract infections. Death from RSV may occur if the patient has other underlying illnesses such as premature respiratory distress syndrome, congenital heart defects, or a compromised immune system.

LABORATORY DIAGNOSIS: Diagnosis is made by culture of respiratory specimens in susceptible cell cultures, direct examination of respiratory specimens for virus-infected cells by immunofluorescence, or detection of virus antigens by ELISA testing.

PREVENTION AND TREATMENT: Mother's milk contains antibodies that neutralize viral activity and this is probably why RSV viral infections are more common in non-breast fed infants. A high percentage of adults tested have antibodies to RSV. These antibodies are not as common in younger children. Infection with RSV does not confer long lasting protection against subsequent reinfection. Ribavirin is used as an effective treatment. No vaccines are available.

Reye's Syndrome described by R. D. K. Reye, in Australia, 1963

DEFINITION: A medical condition characterized by sudden loss of consciousness, and is a serious complication of influenza; occurs mainly in children with influenza B who have taken aspirin.

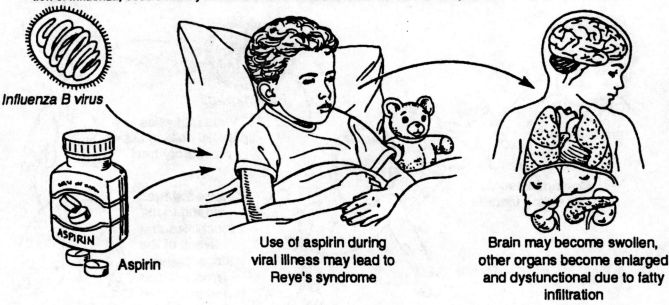

Influenza B virus

Aspirin

Use of aspirin during viral illness may lead to Reye's syndrome

Brain may become swollen, other organs become enlarged and dysfunctional due to fatty infiltration

DESCRIPTION: Reye's syndrome typically follows a case of influenza 3 to 21 days after infection. Although the etiology of this syndrome is largely unknown, there is a strong correlation between the incidence of the disease and certain chemicals in the body, particularly from salicylates or common aspirin when used during a viral illness. Reye's syndrome occurs in clusters during influenza epidemics. Three hundred cases, for example, were diagnosed during an influenza B epidemic in the U.S. in 1973–74. Single cases of Reye's syndrome have also been known to follow infection with varicella-zoster virus, that causes chicken pox, and Epstein-Barr virus (EBV), that causes mononucleosis. The liver and the brain are generally the organs most severely affected. The liver becomes enlarged, and small, fatty droplets accumulate in the cytoplasm of the hepatocytes (liver cells). Fatty infiltration may also damage the kidneys, heart, pancreas, and lungs. The tissue of the brain, on the other hand, becomes swollen without fatty infiltration, and the size of the ventricles is reduced.

SIGNS AND SYMPTOMS: Fever and repeated, severe vomiting are the initial symptoms of Reye's syndrome. Over a period of hours, this may progress to delirium, convulsions, coma, and eventually death. The mortality rate for Reye's syndrome ranges from 5 to 25% in treated cases, and some patients survive without permanent neurological deficits. In comatosed patients with Reye's syndrome, death is almost certain.

PREVENTION AND TREATMENT: Avoiding influenza infection reduces the risk of acquiring Reye's syndrome (see card on Influenza, #197), and vaccines are available for that purpose. Aspirin or salicylate should never be given to a young patient with influenza. No specific cure exists for Reye's syndrome, so treatment is directed at stabilizing the patient's condition and regulating intracranial pressure.

Rheumatic Fever *Gk. rheumatikos,* subject to flux (flow)

DEFINITION: A late sequela of infection with *Streptococcus pyogenes* due to or resulting from two to three weeks of untreated pharyngitis. The *Streptococcus pyogenes* bacteria are usually transmitted through respiratory droplets.

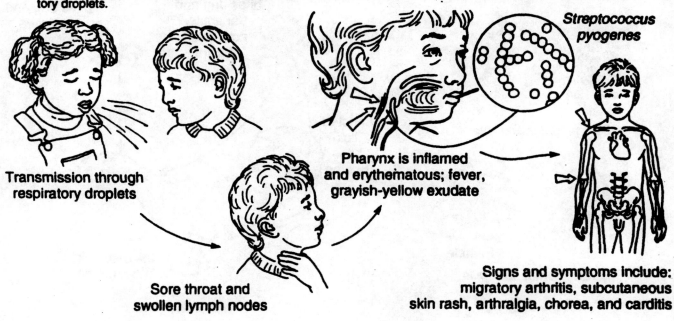

Transmission through respiratory droplets

Sore throat and swollen lymph nodes

Pharynx is inflamed and erythematous; fever, grayish-yellow exudate

Streptococcus pyogenes

Signs and symptoms include: migratory arthritis, subcutaneous skin rash, arthralgia, chorea, and carditis

DESCRIPTION: Rheumatic fever is a nonsuppurative inflammation reaction that may follow infection with *Streptococcus pyogenes,* a gram-positive beta-hemolytic streptococcus. Though the pathogenesis of rheumatic fever is not completely understood, antibodies to the antigens on group A streptococci seem to crossreact with antigens on joint and cardiac tissue. This immunologic reaction usually causes only minor injury to joints but can permanently damage heart valves. Following a severe pharyngeal infection with *Streptococcus pyogenes,* a Type III hypersensitivity reaction takes place causing *Aschoff bodies* to form in the heart valves and cardiac muscle. Destruction of the heart valves creates heart murmurs and damage to the heart muscles reduces the capabilities of heart contractions. Rheumatic valvular heart disease is responsible for approximately 15,000 deaths in the U.S. each year.

SIGNS AND SYMPTOMS: In streptococcal pharyngitis (strep throat), the pharynx is erythematous, contains grayish-yellow exudates, and may bleed when swabbed. Rheumatic fever is usually characterized by high fever, migratory arthritis, and a subcutaneous skin rash, called *erythema marginatum.* Rheumatic fever is also accompanied by arthralgia, chorea, and carditis.

LABORATORY DIAGNOSIS: Aside from the clinical manifestations of rheumatic fever, diagnosis is made by the demonstration of a preceding streptococcal infection, presence of anti-streptolysin O, and the presence of C-reactive protein, and electrocardiographic changes.

PREVENTION AND TREATMENT: Early detection of strep throat infection and treatment with benzathine penicillin is important to prevent rheumatic fever. Most cases of *streptococcal pharyngitis,* however, resolve spontaneously. Since *streptococcal pharyngitis* infection is easily treated, 3% of epidemic and only 0.1% of nonepidemic streptococcal infections in the U.S. lead to rheumatic fever. Rheumatic fever is much more common in developing countries. Rheumatic fever is treated with salicylates or corticosteroids to reduce cardiac and joint inflammation. Monthly administration of penicillin G usually prevents rheumatic recurrence.

Rocky Mountain Spotted Fever

DEFINITION: A tick-borne human rickettsial disease that occurs in parts of North America; caused by *Rickettsia rickettsii*.

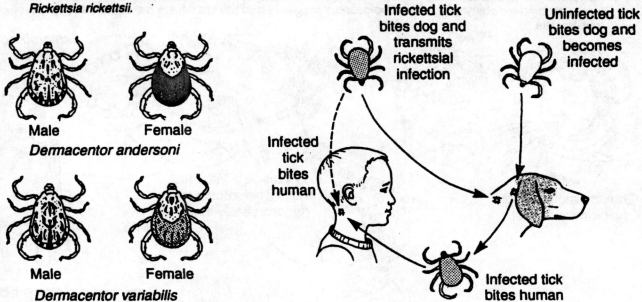

Male   Female
Dermacentor andersoni

Male   Female
Dermacentor variabilis

Tick vectors

Infected tick bites dog and transmits rickettsial infection

Uninfected tick bites dog and becomes infected

Infected tick bites human

Infected tick bites human

Infection cycle

DESCRIPTION: Rocky Mountain spotted fever (RMSF) is contracted from the bite of a tick infected with the causative organism, *Rickettsia rickettsii*. In the western United States, the wood tick, *Dermacentor andersoni*, is the arthropod vector, whereas the dog tick, *Dermacentor variabilis*, is the vector in the eastern United States. Rickettsiae can pass from one generation of ticks to the next through tick eggs—a process called *transovarian passage*. Therefore, mammalian reservoir hosts are not necessary for the reproduction of the rickettsiae. RMSF does not harm ticks, and an estimated 3% of ticks are infected. There are about 650 human cases of RMSF reported in the U.S. each year.

SIGNS AND SYMPTOMS: Rickettsias proliferate in the endothelia of small blood vessels and capillaries. The disease is characterized by fever, malaise, severe headache, and skin rash that appears first on the wrists and palms, and ankles and soles. The incubation period is generally 3 to 12 days. If untreated, the mortality rate is about 5%, generally during the second week of illness.

LABORATORY DIAGNOSIS: A four-fold rise in antibody titer detected in paired sera is diagnostic of this infection. A convalescent serum having a high antibody titer is also considered diagnostic.

PREVENTION AND TREATMENT: The best method of prevention is to avoid being bitten by ticks when camping or hiking in endemic areas. Wearing protective clothing and using arthropod repellents are advisable. It is also important to inspect clothing and the entire body surface for the presence of ticks following campouts or picnics in locations known to be infested with ticks. Ticks should be removed by grasping them with fine tweezers at the point of attachment to the skin and pulling slowly and steadily. The bite should then be cleansed. Ticks should not be removed with bare hands or crushed between the fingers. An attached tick that is infected can be removed within about four hours without causing RMSF because of the necessary *rejuvenation period*. Treatment of RMSF with chloramphenicol or tetracyclines is effective if started early in the illness, and immunity after recovery appears to be permanent.

Rubella (roo-bel'la) L. *rubellus*, reddish

DEFINITION: An acute, infectious disease typically manifest in small children. It is caused by the *rubella virus* which is an enveloped icosahedral RNA *togavirus;* also known as *German measles.*

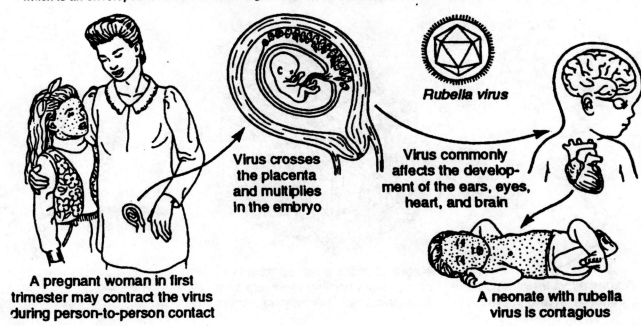

Rubella virus

Virus crosses the placenta and multiplies in the embryo

Virus commonly affects the development of the ears, eyes, heart, and brain

A pregnant woman in first trimester may contract the virus during person-to-person contact

A neonate with rubella virus is contagious

DESCRIPTION: Rubella is the most benign of all childhood communicable diseases. The rubella virus is transmitted by respiratory droplets from person to person. The incubation period is 12 to 23 days. The rubella viruses invade most of the body tissues and can be recovered from the blood, throat, stools, and cerebrospinal fluid. The infection is highly contagious as viruses are shed from the throat of an infected person several days before and after the appearance of the rash. The major danger with the rubella virus is manifest when a woman in the first trimester of pregnancy contracts the disease. The virus crosses the placenta during the viremic stage and multiplies in the cells of an embryo causing chromosomal breakage and interfering with mitosis. More than 40% of such cases result in severe fetal malformations or death. The fetal deformity, called *congenital rubella syndrome,* may affect the eyes (myopia, cataracts, glaucoma), ears (deafness), heart (patent ductus arteriosus), and brain (mental retardation, microcephaly, behavior disorders). A test for immunity to the virus is performed routinely on pregnant women with no cause for concern if their antibody titer is sufficiently high.

SIGNS AND SYMPTOMS: Approximately 30% of the rubella cases are asymptomatic. In the other 70% of the cases, the disease manifests symptoms similar to a common cold. In addition, there may be a mild rash, moderate fever, sore throat, and swollen lymph nodes.

LABORATORY DIAGNOSIS: Diagnosis is made using ELISA tests or the hemagglutination inhibition test (HI test) to detect anti-rubella IgM antibodies or seroconversion.

PREVENTION AND TREATMENT: A live virus rubella vaccine is available in the mumps-measles-rubella combination vaccine (MMR) and is recommended for all healthy children. Non-pregnant women of reproductive age without proof of immunization should be immunized and should avoid pregnancy for three months following the vaccination. The HI test or ELISA test assesses immunity. Natural infection confers life-long immunity in most people, however, re-infections are possible. Treatment is toward management of symptoms. Therapeutic abortions may be recommended in some extreme cases.

Scalded Skin Syndrome

DEFINITION: A rare staphylococcal skin infection that causes necrosis of the epidermal layer of the skin so that it peels off in sheets; also called *Ritter's disease* or *bullous impetigo*.

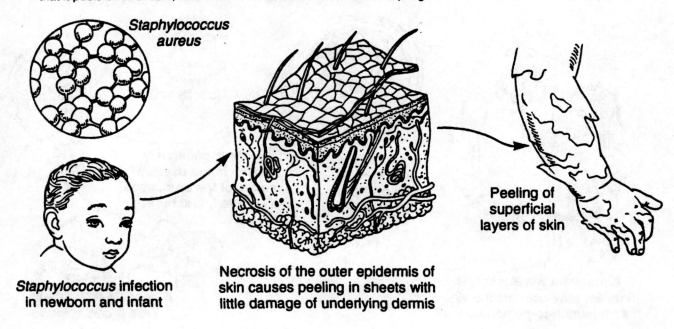

Staphylococcus aureus

Staphylococcus infection in newborn and infant

Necrosis of the outer epidermis of skin causes peeling in sheets with little damage of underlying dermis

Peeling of superficial layers of skin

DESCRIPTION: There are two forms of scalded skin syndrome, the infant form and the adult form. The infant form is a spreading staphylococcal infection that has a predilection for newborns and very young children. As much as 80% of the skin surface may be affected. Although the first layer of skin is destroyed, there is relatively little damage to the underlying dermis. Desquamation, redness, and tenderness of the skin develops in 36 to 48 hours and the patient may be ill with fever, malaise, and anorexia. This disease is caused by an exotoxin of phage Group II coagulase-positive penicillin-resistant staphylococci. In adults, large flaccid blisters appear with full-blown disease occurring in several days.

SIGNS AND SYMPTOMS: First, large bullae form on the skin surface, frequently around the nose or ears, and then the outer skin layer peels off in sheets. The characteristic appearance of this disease gives it the name of "scalded skin syndrome." It looks very much like a large, general burn. The risk of fatal microbial invasion of the lungs or septicemia is always present.

LABORATORY DIAGNOSIS: Bacteriologic culture detects staphylococci in the skin and often in the nasopharynx. Culture also detects secondary septicemic and pulmonary infections. Differentiation of scalded skin syndrome from viral exanthems and drug allergies is important.

PREVENTION AND TREATMENT: Supportive therapy can help to relieve symptoms. Aggressive treatment should be immediately instigated with antibiotics (cloxacillin or methicillin). Corticosteroids are given as the severity warrants and if allergic reactions are suspected. Fluid and electrolyte balance may require correction.

Scarlet Fever L. *scarlatum*, bright red cloth

DEFINITION: Scarlet fever is caused by *Streptococcus pyogenes*, the bacterium responsible for streptococcal pharyngitis. Though the infection is localized in the oropharynx and upper respiratory tract, its exotoxins cause a diffuse red rash on the neck, torso, and extremities.

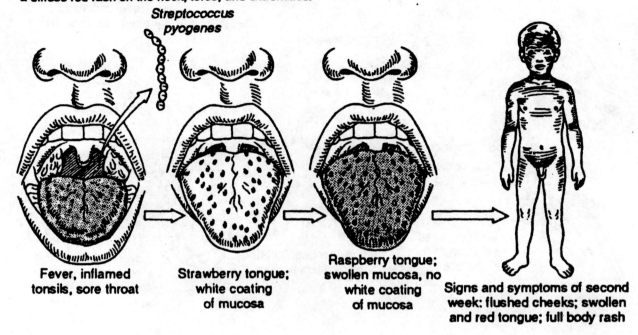

Streptococcus pyogenes

Fever, inflamed tonsils, sore throat

Strawberry tongue; white coating of mucosa

Raspberry tongue; swollen mucosa, no white coating of mucosa

Signs and symptoms of second week: flushed cheeks; swollen and red tongue; full body rash

DESCRIPTION: *Streptococcus pyogenes* is a gram-positive beta-hemolytic streptococcus, that is transmitted by airborne respiratory droplets to the oropharynx and upper respiratory tract. A sore throat, headache, malaise, nausea, and high fever follow a short incubation period. This is followed by a "strawberry" tongue and a "raspberry" tongue, and then a diffuse erythematous rash on the neck, trunk, and extremities. The rash is caused by the release of erythrogenic exotoxin from lysogenized bacteria. The rash is perifollicular, edematous, and bumpy, almost like coarse sandpaper. It begins on the neck and trunk, and within hours spreads all over the body except around the mouth. The incidence of scarlet fever has progressively declined in the U.S. and most European countries. It remains a problem as a childhood disease in developing countries and mortality is high when seriously ill patients are not treated with antibiotics.

SIGNS AND SYMPTOMS: High fever, swollen cervical lymph nodes, enlarged tonsils, sore throat, and characteristic strawberry and raspberry appearance of the tongue are early symptoms of scarlet fever. The erythemic rash that fades when thumb pressure is applied is characteristic of the later stage of the disease. Mild cases of scarlet fever are frequently referred to as *scarlatina*.

LABORATORY DIAGNOSIS: Scarlet fever is diagnosed by laboratory culture. Several rapid direct specimen tests exist for the diagnosis of infection in the physician's office. These tests, however, should be performed only with standard culture backup tests because of their relatively low sensitivity.

PREVENTION AND TREATMENT: Since *Streptococcus pyogenes* is spread by contact with an infectious person, care should be taken to avoid exposure. Early detection of scarlet fever infection and treatment with benzathine penicillin, penicillin G, penicillin V, or sulfadiazine is important in establishing a quick resolution to the disease. Most infections of *Streptococcal pharyngitis*, however, resolve themselves.

Sindbis Fever

DEFINITION: A viral disease commonly found in Africa, Asia, Scandinavia, and The Commonwealth of Independent States, caused by the *Sindbis virus*, a member of the genus *Alphavirus* in the *Togavirus* family. It is transmitted between bird hosts and between birds and humans by the mosquito vector, *Culex*.

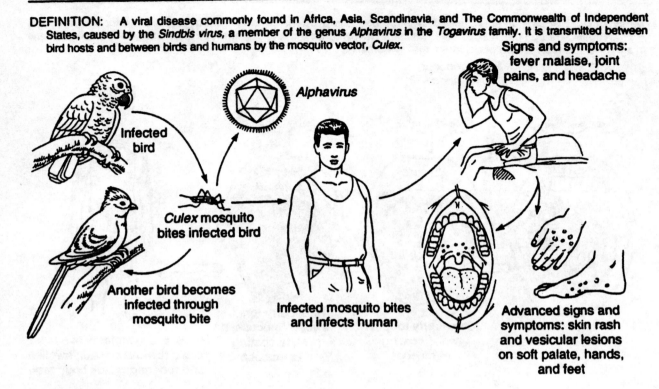

Signs and symptoms: fever malaise, joint pains, and headache

Alphavirus

Infected bird

Culex mosquito bites infected bird

Another bird becomes infected through mosquito bite

Infected mosquito bites and infects human

Advanced signs and symptoms: skin rash and vesicular lesions on soft palate, hands, and feet

DESCRIPTION: A number of wild bird species are affected with the viral pathogen of this disease. *Culex* mosquitoes transfer the disease between birds and can also infect humans with their bite. Most cases are related to the mosquito density and human exposure in rural areas. The disease is largely confined to isolated areas of Africa, Australia, Asia, and the Middle East. The *Sindbis virus* is a prominent model for the study of virus structure and gene expression of *Alphaviruses*.

SIGNS AND SYMPTOMS: The incubation period for sindbis fever is 3–6 days. It begins with an abrupt onset of fever, malaise, joint pains, and headache. These symptoms are followed by a papular rash, small vesicular lesions on the soft palate, and larger vesicular lesions on the hands and the feet. The virus can be isolated from these lesions. Most patients recover in a week, but some patients may have localized arthritis in the joints of the hands and feet which may persist for many weeks. Uncommon complications include encephalitis and myocarditis. Sindbis fever is usually milder in children than in adults.

LABORATORY DIAGNOSIS: Diagnosis is made by demonstrating an antibody rise in convalescent-phase serum compared to acute-phase serum. Immunofluorescence, hemagglutination inhibition, complement fixation, or virus neutralization tests are used. Virus isolation from cerebrospinal fluid is rarely successful.

PREVENTION AND TREATMENT: Avoiding rural areas heavily infested with mosquitoes and also avoiding mosquito bites through the use of protective netting and insect repellents are preventative measures for sindbis fever. Ribavirin has been reported to inhibit this virus. No vaccine is available for sindbis fever, however, antipyretics and analgesics may be used to manage the disease because it is self-limiting. Intravenous fluids may be needed for adequate hydration.

Smallpox Anglo Saxon: *smael*, tiny; *poc*, pustule

DEFINITION: An acute, highly communicable febrile disease caused by the variola virus, a *poxvirus*, and characterized by the appearance of skin eruptions, severe pyrexia, and backache. Smallpox is considered to have been eradicated worldwide; also called *variola*.

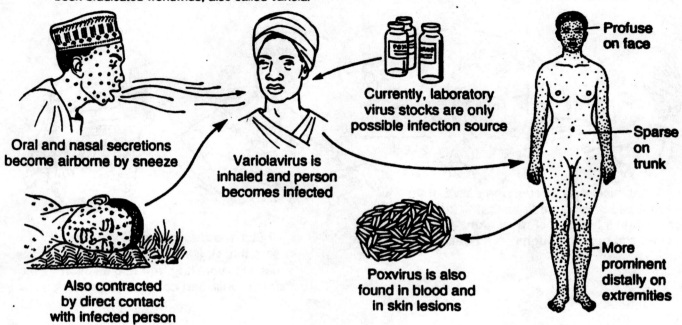

Oral and nasal secretions become airborne by sneeze

Also contracted by direct contact with infected person

Variolavirus is inhaled and person becomes infected

Currently, laboratory virus stocks are only possible infection source

Poxvirus is also found in blood and in skin lesions

Profuse on face

Sparse on trunk

More prominent distally on extremities

DESCRIPTION: Although eradicated worldwide, smallpox has produced fearsome scourges throughout history. A discussion of smallpox is now of more historic than practical interest. The variola virus would enter a victim's body through the respiratory tract and was transferred to other people by buccal and nasal secretions. The virus was also found in the patient's blood and skin lesions. It remained active for a long time in the dried crusts of skin lesions. Even the dead bodies of victims were dangerous sources of infection. The last naturally occurring case of smallpox was reported in Somalia, East Africa in 1977 and the eradication of smallpox is regarded as a great triumph of 20th century medicine. Eradication was possible because humans are the only hosts of the disease, asymptomatic carriage and latent infection did not occur, and there was an effective vaccine in existence. Furthermore, the disease could be relatively easily diagnosed, and the virus was genetically stable with few mutants. Smallpox could now only reappear if laboratory stocks of poxviruses were released or if animal poxviruses mutated to human virulence.

SIGNS AND SYMPTOMS: An increased fever and severe constitutional signs and symptoms were the initial symptoms. A rash then appeared most profuse on the face and distally on the arms and legs. It was relatively sparse on the trunk. Death frequently resulted from the overwhelming primary viral infection or from bacterial superinfection. Smallpox victims who did survive frequently had disfiguring scars from the healed lesions.

LABORATORY DIAGNOSIS: Clinical diagnosis was confirmed by detecting antibody rises in convalescent sera or isolation of variola virus from the serous fluid of the skin lesions.

PREVENTION AND TREATMENT: An immunization consisting of a live virus vaccine (the vaccinia virus) is available although it is no longer thought to be necessary to distribute the vaccine since smallpox is considered to be eradicated. A population of the poxvirus is maintained in two reference laboratories, one in Atlanta, Georgia, and one in Moscow, Russia.

DEFINITION: Common bacterial infection generally in school-aged children whose primary symptom is a sore throat; also known as *streptococcal pharyngitis*.

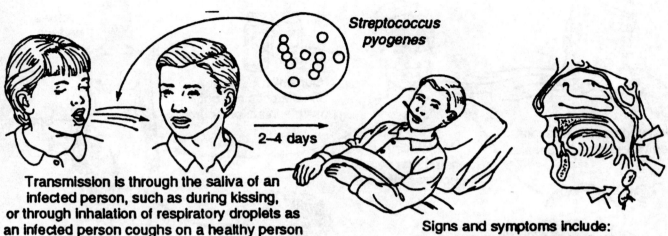

Streptococcus pyogenes

2–4 days

Transmission is through the saliva of an infected person, such as during kissing, or through inhalation of respiratory droplets as an infected person coughs on a healthy person

Signs and symptoms include: sore throat, fever, abdominal pain, nausea, vomiting, red and swollen pharynx, enlarged cervical lymph nodes

DESCRIPTION: Strep throat is generally caused by group A beta-hemolytic streptococci, known as *Streptococcus pyogenes*. Group C and G streptococci may occasionally be involved. Streptococci are spherical or ovoid bacteria, 0.6 to 1.0 μm in diameter, that grow in chains of varying lengths. They are aerotolerant, gram-positive, nonspore-forming, and nonmotile. These bacteria are classified by the way they hemolyze erythrocytes on blood agar plates (beta hemolytic) and by cell-wall antigens (group A, B, etc.). Strep throat occurs primarily in children 5 to 15 years of age, although all age groups are susceptible. The bacteria are spread by person-to-person contact via droplets of saliva or nasal secretions. The normal incubation period is 2 to 4 days. Rheumatic fever or scarlet fever may follow pharyngeal streptococcus infection. In the latter case, streptococci elaborate erythrogenic toxin which causes the rash characteristic of scarlet fever.

SIGNS AND SYMPTOMS: Abrupt onset of sore throat accompanied by malaise, fever of 101° F to 104° F, and headache. Nausea, vomiting, and abdominal pain are common in children. The pharynx appears red and swollen, and lymph nodes beneath the jaw become enlarged and tender. Strep throat is usually self-limiting. The fever abates in 3 to 5 days, and virtually all acute symptoms subside within one week.

LABORATORY DIAGNOSIS: Diagnosis is commonly made by obtaining a throat specimen and allowing the bacteria to grow in culture. Several rapid direct antigen tests are available for in-office testing, but they lack the sensitivity of culture. It is thought that sole dependence on the rapid tests for diagnosis is leading to a resurgence of scarlet fever and rheumatic fever.

PREVENTION AND TREATMENT: Other members of the family or other persons should have limited contact with the patient to minimize the chance of spreading the infection, and tissue paper soiled with nasal secretions should be properly disposed. Treatment is directed toward prevention of such complications as acute rheumatic fever or acute sinusitis. Penicillin or erythromycin are the drugs of choice for accomplishing this, and the antibiotics should be continued for a full 10 days after diagnosis.

Superficial Mycoses Gk. *mykes*, fungus; *osis*, condition

DEFINITION: Any fungus skin disease occurring on various parts of the body and named according to the body part affected; caused by a variety of dermatophytes, or fungal parasites of the skin.

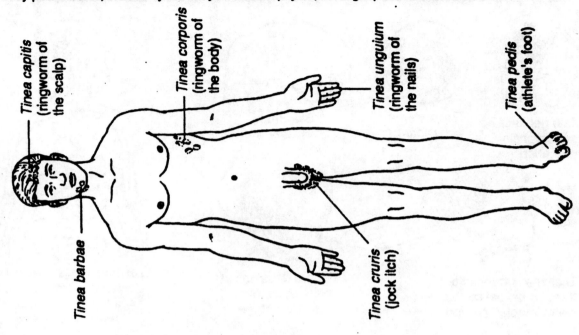

DESCRIPTION: Fungal infections of the skin, nails, and hair are common and most are very contagious. The most commonly involved genera are *Microsporum*, *Trichophyton*, and *Epidermophyton*. *Tinea capitis* (scalp ringworm) is an infection of the scalp and hair, caused by *Microsporum* and *Trichophyton* and most frequently afflicts children. *Tinea corporis* (ringworm of the body), caused by *Trichophyton*, affects the trunk and arms producing red, slightly elevated patches, and causing considerable itching. *Tinea cruris* (jock itch) is infection of the surfaces of the crural, anal, and genital areas. *Tinea barbae* is a fungal infection of the bearded portions of the neck and face. *Tinea pedis* (athlete's foot) is an infection of the feet. It is generally not acquired from lockerroom floors, but rather, shoes that are not well ventilated and socks that do not absorb moisture create the environment for the fungus to grow. *Tinea unguium* (ringworm of the nails) is caused by *Trichophyton spp.*

SIGNS AND SYMPTOMS: Although each of the mycoses have particular symptoms, the general indications of a fungal infection includes scaling, slight itching, and reddish or grayish patches. Hair will become dry and brittle and is easily extracted from the hair follicle. If the infection moves deeper, then flat, reddish tumors may appear containing dead or broken hairs and gaping follicular orifices. Pus may also be discharged through dilated follicular openings. Moist environments, such as on the feet, encourage bacterial growth which produces white, soggy, patches of malodorous skin and itching between the toes.

LABORATORY DIAGNOSIS: Diagnosis is made by demonstration of fungus in scrapings of lesions either by direct microscopic examination or by culture.

PREVENTION AND TREATMENT: Personal hygiene is very important in preventing and controlling mycoses. The feet should be dried carefully after bathing, especially between the toes. Affected persons should not allow personal items such as clothes, towels, combs, and sports equipment to be used by others. Griseofulvin is the antimicrobial agent given orally for all types of superficial mycoses. Topical preparations containing fungicidal agents are useful in treatment of the superficial mycoses, however, recurrences are frequent.

Syphilis (sif'i-lis) *Syphilis* -shepherd having the disease in a Latin poem

DEFINITION: An infectious, chronic, generally sexually or congenitally transmitted disease; affecting any tissue or vascular organ; may persist for years without symptoms; caused by the spirochete *Treponema pallidum.*

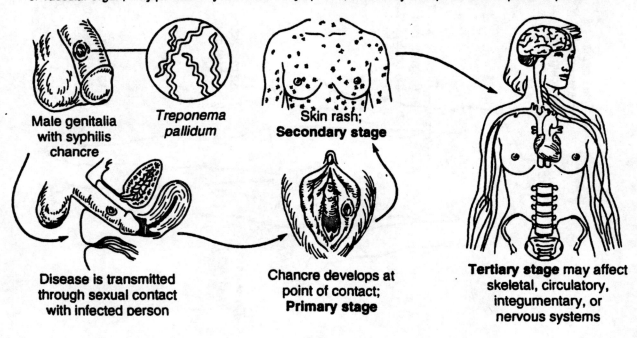

Male genitalia with syphilis chancre

Treponema pallidum

Skin rash; **Secondary stage**

Disease is transmitted through sexual contact with infected person

Chancre develops at point of contact; **Primary stage**

Tertiary stage may affect skeletal, circulatory, integumentary, or nervous systems

DESCRIPTION: Syphilis is generally a sexually transmitted disease but it can also be contracted by transfusion of infected blood or plasma, from mother to fetus, or as an accidental laboratory infection. Transmission may also occur by anal-rectal contact, fellatio, and occasionally by kissing. The syphilis spirochete usually enters through the skin or mucous membranes.

SIGNS AND SYMPTOMS: The symptoms are described in three stages. During the *primary stage,* a *chancre* develops at the location of the portal of spirochete entry. The chancre is an ulcerated sore that has hard edges and endures for 10 days to 3 months. The chancre will heal with time, but if the disease is not treated, the primary stage may be followed by the secondary and tertiary stages of syphilis. During the primary stage, the bacteria may enter the bloodstream and spread throughout the body. The *secondary stage* of syphilis is expressed by lesions or a rash of the skin and mucous membranes, accompanied by fever. This stage lasts from 2 weeks to 6 months, and the symptoms disappear of their own accord. Syphilis is highly contagious during the primary and secondary stages. The *tertiary stage* occurs 10 to 20 years following primary infection. The circulatory, integumentary, skeletal, and nervous systems are particularly vulnerable to the degenerative changes caused by this disease. The end result of untreated syphilis may be blindness, insanity, and eventually death.

LABORATORY DIAGNOSIS: The spirochetes may be detected in exudates of the lesions by darkfield microscopy. Serological tests include the Venereal Disease Research Laboratory (VDRL) test, the rapid plasma reagin (RPR) test, and the fluorescent treponemal antibody absorption (FTA-ABS) test.

PREVENTION AND TREATMENT: The most effective prevention is through careful partner choice for sexual activity and the practice of "safe sex" with the correct use of condoms. Education of the extensive prevalence and symptoms of syphilis and other sexually transmitted diseases is very important. Infected persons should be identified and treated. There is no vaccine for syphilis, and administration of penicillin is the usual treatment. Other antibiotics can be used in the case of allergic reaction to penicillin. Destruction of tissue that occurs during the tertiary stage cannot be reduced, however, regardless of the treatment. After a patient is cured, no protective immunity exists and reinfection may readily occur.

Tetanus (tet'a-nus) Gk. *tetanos*, stretched

DEFINITION: A disease of humans and other mammals with symptoms resulting from the neurotoxin produced by *Clostridium tetani*, a spore-forming, gram-positive bacillus; also called *lockjaw*.

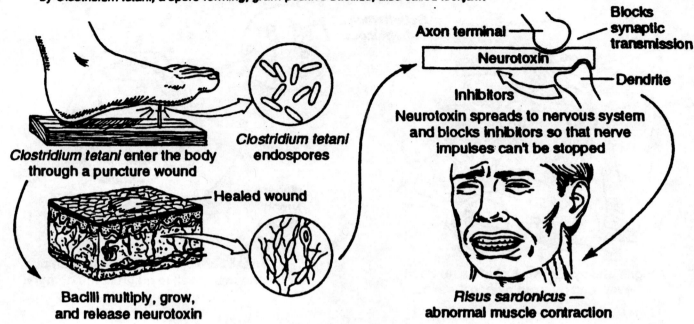

Clostridium tetani enter the body through a puncture wound

Clostridium tetani endospores

Healed wound

Bacilli multiply, grow, and release neurotoxin

Axon terminal

Blocks synaptic transmission

Neurotoxin

Inhibitors

Dendrite

Neurotoxin spreads to nervous system and blocks inhibitors so that nerve impulses can't be stopped

Risus sardonicus — abnormal muscle contraction

DESCRIPTION: Spores of *Clostridium tetani* are abundant in nature and can be introduced into human tissue from the soil or dirty clothing following a cut, abrasion, compound fracture, or puncture wound. The trauma may heal completely before the symptoms of the disease appear. Once within the anaerobic environment of the body, the endospores of *C. tetani* germinate, and the bacilli grow, divide, and release the neurotoxin. The neurotoxin spreads systemically and eventually reaches the central nervous system where it blocks the release of inhibitory impulses. This lack of inhibition causes hyperactivity of motor neurons and spastic muscle paralysis.

SIGNS AND SYMPTOMS: The primary symptom of tetanus is abnormal muscle contraction. The muscles of the jaw and neck are stimulated to contract convulsively so that the mouth remains closed, making swallowing difficult. Other muscles jerk and are thrown into intense and painful contractions lasting from a few seconds to several minutes. This causes the back to arch and the face to have a distinctive tight, unnatural smile known as *risus sardonicus*. If untreated, tetanus is frequently fatal due to respiratory failure or exhaustion. The mortality rate ranges from 30 to 90% depending upon the circumstances of the infection. If the patient does recover, there are no lasting effects.

LABORATORY DIAGNOSIS: Culture is infrequently successful, but in some cases yields *C. tetani* from the wound.

PREVENTION AND TREATMENT: Tetanus is now uncommon in developed nations because the diphtheria-pertussis-tetanus (DPT) vaccine makes the disease preventable. Immunizations should begin at 2 months of age and continue regularly until one year of age. Boosters are needed every ten years thereafter. If a wound occurs, it must be carefully and completely cleaned. Antibiotic therapy (usually penicillin) may also be used, and the administration of tetanus toxoid to boost immunity is standard procedure. Patients with tetanus are frequently treated with muscle relaxants and respiratory assistance. A tracheostomy may also be necessary.

Tonsillitis L. *tonsilla*, almond; *itis*, inflammation

DEFINITION: Inflammation of the tonsils, may be caused by a number of viruses and bacteria.

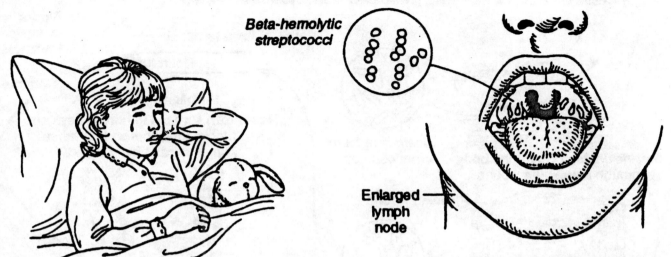

Beta-hemolytic streptococci

Enlarged lymph node

Signs and symptoms include sore throat, fever, and referred pain to the ears

Tonsils are swollen with yellowish pus, and may swell to obstruct the pharynx

DESCRIPTION: The palatine tonsils are masses of lymphatic tissue located in the mucous membranes on both lateral sides of the oropharynx. They act as filters to protect the body from invasions of bacteria entering through the mouth and nose. Tonsillitis results when the tonsils are so overrun with infection that they become the source of infection. This disorder commonly affects children between 5 and 10 years old, and may be acute or chronic in nature. Acute illness generally results from infection with beta-hemolytic streptococci, but it may be caused by other bacteria or viruses. Illness usually lasts 4 to 6 days. Serious complications such as sinusitis, abscesses, or rheumatic fever may occur in conjunction with chronic tonsillitis.

SIGNS AND SYMPTOMS: Acute tonsillitis begins with mild to severe sore throat. A very young child unable to complain about a sore throat may stop eating. Difficulty swallowing, fever reaching 105° F, chills, swelling and tenderness of the lymph glands beneath the jaw, muscle and joint pain, malaise, headache, and referred pain to the ears are common symptoms. The tonsils appear enlarged and red with yellowish discharge, and they hypertrophy and obstruct the pharynx. Chronic illness presents recurring sore throat and purulent drainage from the tonsils.

LABORATORY DIAGNOSIS: Bacteriological diagnosis is made by culture. The isolate is tested for antibiotic sensitivity so effective antibiotic therapy can be instituted.

PREVENTION AND TREATMENT: Little can be done to prevent tonsillitis beyond normal precautions for avoiding colds and infection. Rest, adequate fluid intake, and antibiotics are the most important aspects of treatment. For tonsillitis caused by group A beta-hemolytic streptococcus, penicillin is the drug of choice. Tetracycline and erythromycin are also effective. Antibiotic therapy should continue for 10 days to prevent bacteria from elaborating the toxic substances which cause rheumatic fever. *Tonsillectomy* is the only effective treatment for chronic tonsillitis of the palatine tonsils. *Adenoiditis* is inflammation of the lymphatic pharyngeal tonsils, and an *adenoidectomy* is the surgical removal of the adenoids. Tonsillectomies and adenoidectomies are less common today than they were in the past due to the availability of powerful antibiotics.

Toxic Shock Syndrome

DEFINITION: A rare and sometimes fatal disease caused by a toxin produced by certain strains of *Staphylococcus aureus*. It is contracted predominantly by young women during their first few years of menstruation.

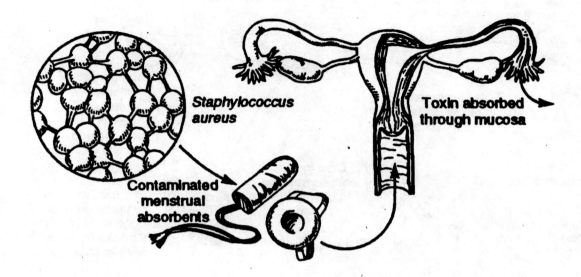

Staphylococcus aureus

Toxin absorbed through mucosa

Contaminated menstrual absorbents

DESCRIPTION: Toxic Shock Syndrome (TSS) is usually associated with an infection with pyrogenic exotoxin-producing lysogenic strains of phage—group I *Staphylococcus aureus*. The organism has been found colonizing the nasopharynx or vagina of affected patients. The toxin involved is toxic shock syndrome toxin-1 (TSST-1). Toxin production is promoted in Mg^{++}-depleted environments. In menstruating women, a tampon provides a favorable environment for growth of the organism and elaboration of the toxin. Superabsorbent tampons are the most dangerous because they are changed less frequently, they allow the build-up of organisms and toxin, and they chelate Mg^{++}.

SIGNS AND SYMPTOMS: The initial symptom of TSS is a sudden high fever (>102° F). This is soon followed by vomiting, diarrhea, hypotension, oliguria and diffuse erythematous rash. Further symptoms include desquamation, particularly of the palms of the hands and soles of the feet. Other possible symptoms are intermittent confusion, headache, blurred vision and purulent vaginal discharge. Complications include respiratory distress, cardiac dysfunction, and abnormal liver function.

LABORATORY DIAGNOSIS: Culture of specimen material may grow *S. aureus*. Antibiotic sensitivity testing of the isolate provides information for choosing an appropriate antibiotic, but therapy should not be delayed.

PREVENTION AND TREATMENT: Washing hands regularly before inserting tampons is an important preventative technique. Super-absorbent tampons should also be avoided and no tampon should ever be left in the vagina for over 12 hours. Removing a tampon at night and using an absorbent pad is one way to reduce the risk of TSS. Treatment of TSS consists of management of shock and renal failure if present by fluid and electrolyte replacement. Beta-lactamase-resistant penicillin or cephalosporin are the most frequently used drugs for treating patients with TSS.

Toxoplasmosis Gk. *toxikon,* poison; *plasma,* something formed

DEFINITION: An acute or chronic disease of humans and other animals caused by the protozoan parasite *Toxoplasma gondii;* transmission occurs by ingesting oocysts from contaminated cat feces or tissue cysts in undercooked meat.

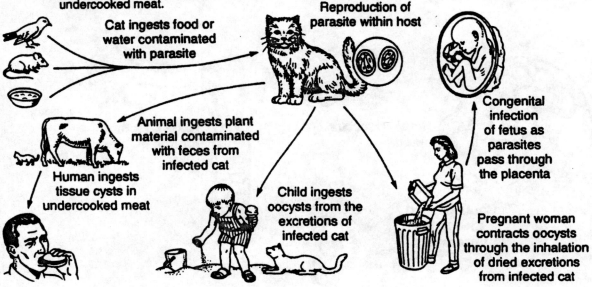

DESCRIPTION: The domestic cat is the most significant host animal in the *Toxoplasma gondii* life cycle. *T. gondii* is the protozoan causative organism of toxoplasmosis. The organism undergoes its only sexual phase in the intestine of the cat, with oocysts eliminated in the cat's feces, thereby contaminating the food or water ingested by other animals. *T. gondii* reproduces asexually in these secondary hosts. The principal modes of human infection are by eating undercooked meat contaminated with the tissue cysts of the parasite and by ingesting directly the oocysts. Inhalation of the dried feces of a cat while cleaning a litter box is also a common mode of contracting the parasite. The parasite can readily pass the placenta of a pregnant woman and congenitally affect the fetus. *T. gondii* is one of the most common causes of central nervous system infection in AIDS patients. It often causes focal or diffuse seizures or changes of mental status.

SIGNS AND SYMPTOMS: Persons with toxoplasmosis are frequently asymptomatic. When symptoms are present, they may mimic pneumonia, hepatitis, myocarditis, or lymphadenitis. Fatigue, chills, fever, and headache are common. Congenital involvement during pregnancy may result in fetal brain and eye damage, lesions of visceral organs, or a spontaneous abortion.

LABORATORY DIAGNOSIS: Diagnosis is based on serologic tests, lymph node histology, the demonstration of trophozoites in body tissues or fluids, or isolation of *T. gondii.* Serologic tests, such as ELISA tests or immunofluorescence tests, detect IgM or IgG antibodies, indicating current or past infections. Detection of IgM in a neonate generally denotes congenital infection.

PREVENTION AND TREATMENT: Because toxoplasmosis is so prevalent in domestic cats, avoidance of them is a safeguard against the disease. Ingested meat should be adequately cooked. Treatment of toxoplasmosis is with pyrimethamine in combination with either trisulfapyrimidines or sulfadiazine.

Travelers' Diarrhea

DEFINITION: Bacterial illness contracted by some travelers visiting countries with inadequate sanitation; generally caused by *Escherichia coli*; also called *Montezuma's revenge*.

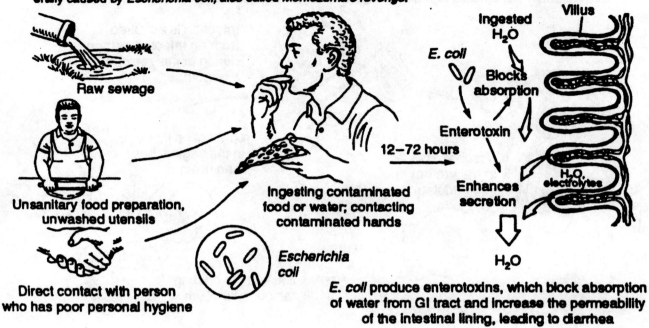

Raw sewage

Unsanitary food preparation, unwashed utensils

Direct contact with person who has poor personal hygiene

Ingesting contaminated food or water; contacting contaminated hands

12–72 hours

Escherichia coli

Ingested H_2O

E. coli

Blocks absorption

Enterotoxin

Enhances secretion

Villus

H_2O, electrolytes

H_2O

E. coli produce enterotoxins, which block absorption of water from GI tract and increase the permeability of the intestinal lining, leading to diarrhea

---

DESCRIPTION: Diarrhea is the travelers' most common malady. This disorder is caused primarily by the bacterium *Escherichia coli*, and occasionally by *Campylobacter* strains. Enteric viruses, such as the Norwalk virus, may also play a role. These organisms are transmitted to humans by food or water contaminated with infected feces. Unsanitary food preparation, unwashed utensils, and dirty hands of another person are also common routes of infection. Following an incubation period of 12 to 72 hours, *E. coli* produces enterotoxins which act on epithelial cells in the mucosa of the small intestine. These substances block resorption of water from the intestine while increasing the permeability of the intestinal lining. This results in an outpouring of fluids and electrolytes. Although illness is normally limited to 3 to 4 days, diarrhea may recur during a single trip, and some *Campylobacter* infections are known to cause chronic, recurring illness. The destination determines the risk to travelers. High-risk countries include most developing countries in Latin America, Africa, the Middle East, and Asia. Southern Europe, and a few Caribbean islands present a moderate risk.

SIGNS AND SYMPTOMS: A tourist with travelers' diarrhea will generally experience four to six loose or watery stools daily. Nausea and vomiting, abdominal cramps, malaise, fever, and occasionally bloody stools may accompany diarrhea.

PREVENTION AND TREATMENT: Changes in eating habits are usually effective means of prevention. Travelers should always wash hands before eating. Fresh, unpeeled vegetables and fruit, raw meat, and raw seafood should be eliminated from the diet. Travelers should drink only bottled water and other bottled beverages, avoiding ice, cold teas, and unpasteurized dairy products. In treatment, fluid and electrolyte loss can usually be balanced by drinking fruit juices, soft drinks without caffeine, and salted crackers. Charcoal, bismuth, and *Lactobacillus* preparations are widely used in alleviating diarrhea, as antimotility and antimicrobial agents. Patients with severe dehydration need oral rehydration with solutions of water and electrolytes. Antibiotics are not usually needed except in cases of severe or prolonged illness.

Trichomoniasis (trik-o-mo-ni'ah-sis) Gk. *trich*, hair; *monas*, single unit

DEFINITION: A sexually transmitted infection of the male and female reproductive tracts caused by the flagellated protozoan *Trichomonas vaginalis*, giving rise to vaginitis or urethritis.

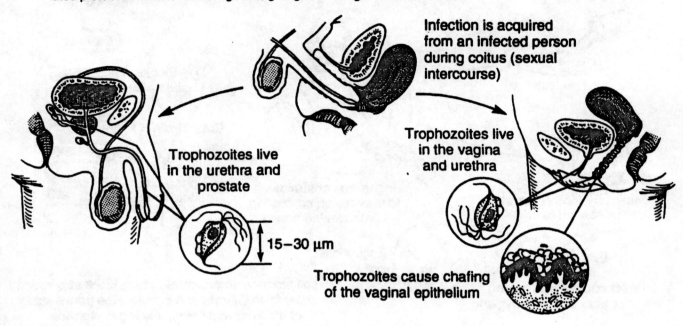

DESCRIPTION: Trichomoniasis is contracted by having coitus (sexual intercourse) with a person who is infected with *Trichomonas vaginalis* protozoa. It is one of the most common sexually transmitted diseases, and in most areas of the U.S. the incidence among tested females is 25 to 30 percent. In a warm and moist environment, the trophozoite can survive for a few hours outside of the body. In females, the vagina is the usual site of trichomoniasis, but in a chronic infection the urethra is also infected. In males, the urethra and prostate are the sites of infection. *T. vaginalis* is a pear-shaped protozoan. It has a single *nucleus*, an *axostyle*, an *undulating membrane*, and four *flagella* that permit movement in quick, jerky rotations. There is no cyst stage in this protozoan and trichomoniasis is, therefore, essentially a sexually transmitted disease.

SIGNS AND SYMPTOMS: Infection in a female is accompanied by pruritis (itching) of the vulva, vaginal stinging, soreness of the perineum and thighs, and a burning sensation during urination. There is also a yellowish vaginal discharge. Males are frequently asymptomatic, and may be unknowing hosts of the disease. In approximately one-half of the infected males, however, there is discomfort in the urethra and pain during urination. A transient purulent urethral discharge may be present.

LABORATORY DIAGNOSIS: Wet mounts of the specimen are observed for trophozoites under dark field or bright field microscopy. Also, media may be inoculated and observed for growth of the protozoan.

PREVENTION AND TREATMENT: Careful partner choice for sexual activity and the use of condoms reduces the chance of infection. Metronidazole is an effective drug treatment of infected persons, as well as tinidazole and miconazole.

Tuberculosis (tu-ber''ku-lo'sis) Gk. *tuberculum*, a swelling; *osis*, condition

DEFINITION: An infectious respiratory disease caused by the tubercle bacillus, *Mycobacterium tuberculosis;* characterized by the formation of tubercles which eventually cause cell necrosis; also called *TB.*

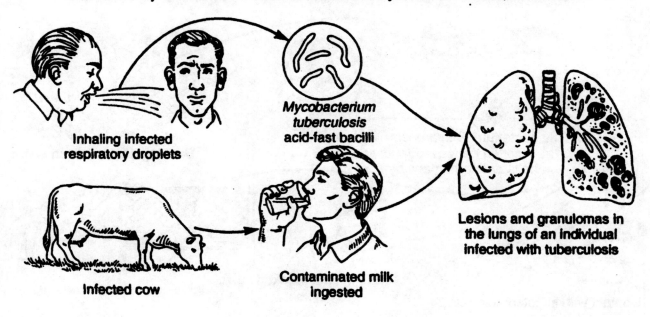

Inhaling infected
respiratory droplets

*Mycobacterium
tuberculosis*
acid-fast bacilli

Infected cow

Contaminated milk
ingested

Lesions and granulomas in
the lungs of an individual
infected with tuberculosis

DESCRIPTION: A tuberculosis (TB) infection is usually acquired through contact with an infected person, but it can also occur by drinking unpasteurized, contaminated milk from an infected cow. The most frequent mode of contraction is through the respiratory system as inhaled microorganisms enter the lungs and penetrate the alveoli. Alveolar macrophages are able to phagocytize most inhaled pathogens, but the bacteria are able to grow within the host's cells. If the bacilli are able to enter the lymphatic system, they actively multiply, causing tissue destruction and the formation of lesions. Granulomas develop as defensive cells surround the lesions. Tissue destruction is mediated largely by the delayed hypersensitivity response. TB may be restricted to the area of primary lesions and granulomas, or it may also spread into other body locations including bones, joints, peritoneum, and urinary and reproductive organs. Malnutrition is a factor in the susceptibility to TB and its course of development. Active TB is an important secondary infection in AIDS patients.

SIGNS AND SYMPTOMS: An infection may be outwardly asymptomatic. When tubercles grow and spread, however, the patient experiences fever, fatigue, weight loss and a cough. As more damage occurs in the lungs, severe dyspnea and chest pain become prominent. Whether an infection results in pathology depends on the number of bacilli present, their virulence, and the resistance of the subject. If untreated, 50% of TB patients die within a two year period.

LABORATORY DIAGNOSIS: The *tine test* is used to identify the presence of infection in which a small amount of bacterial antigen, called *tuberculin,* is injected into the skin. A skin reaction typical of the delayed hypersensitivity response indicates a positive result. Cultures of sputum may reveal tubercle bacilli, but the generation time of the organism is long and positive cultures require a long time to develop. Regular chest radiographs are recommended for individuals whose work brings them into close contact with active cases.

PREVENTION AND TREATMENT: The sputum of infected individuals should be avoided. Infected sputum should not be allowed to dry or infectious organisms could become airborne. TB can be arrested if host resistance mechanisms are active and if antimicrobials are given. Chemotherapeutic agents, such as isoniazid, streptomycin, and rifampin, are also quite effective in stopping the spread of disease, but must be administered over a long period of time. BCG vaccine to control tuberculosis is used in a few countries, but not in the U.S.

Tularemia (tu-lar-e'me-a) Tulare county, California where discovered

DEFINITION: An acute, infectious disease of wild rabbits and rodents caused by the bacterium, *Francisella tularensis;* also known as *rabbit fever.*

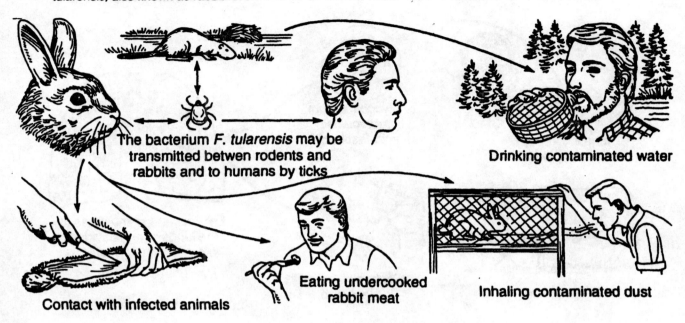

The bacterium *F. tularensis* may be transmitted betwen rodents and rabbits and to humans by ticks

Drinking contaminated water

Contact with infected animals

Eating undercooked rabbit meat

Inhaling contaminated dust

DESCRIPTION: Tularemia is caused by the bacterium, *Francisella tularensis,* and can be transmitted from animal to animal through vector insect bites. *F. tularensis* is a small, pleomorphic, non-motile, non-sporulating, aerobic bacillus. It is transmitted to man by the bite of an infected tick, or other bloodsucking insect; by direct contact with infected animals, or through apparently unbroken skin; by eating inadequately cooked meat, or by drinking water that contains the infectious bacterium. Inhalation of bacilli is a possible route of infection. The bacteria become intracellular parasites in phagocytic cells. Tularemia is a fairly rare disease with fewer than 200 cases per year in the U.S., however due to the severity of the disease and the many modes of infection, it is considered serious.

SIGNS AND SYMPTOMS: Headache, chilliness, vomiting, aching pains, and fever develop about three days after the infection. The site of infection frequently develops into an ulcer. Lymph nodes at the elbow or in the armpit become enlarged, tender, and painful and may later become abscessed. There is sweating, loss of weight and debility. The infection may assume a form of septicemia and result in death. Disseminated necrotic lesions may be found in various body sites. In nonfatal cases, convalescence is slow.

LABORATORY DIAGNOSIS: Diagnosis is made through culture of the organism recovered from lesions, lymph nodes, or sputum. Because *F. tularensis* is so infectious, culture isolation should be attempted only in appropriate protective hoods. Agglutination tests are used to demonstrate a rising antibody titer.

PREVENTION AND TREATMENT: Since infection is associated with rabbits, rodents, and insect bites, tick and fly bites should be avoided and wild animals that seem ill or that are mysteriously dead should not be handled. An attack of tularemia is followed by life-long immunity. Vaccination is available and indicated for those at risk. Treatment is effective using streptomycin or gentamycin.

Typhoid Fever (ti'foyd) Gk. *typhos*, fever; *eidos*, form, shape

DEFINITION: An acute infectious disease characterized by prolonged fever, abdominal rose spots, diarrhea, abdominal pain, and splenomegaly. Typhoid fever is caused by the *Salmonella typhi* bacillus and occurs only in humans.

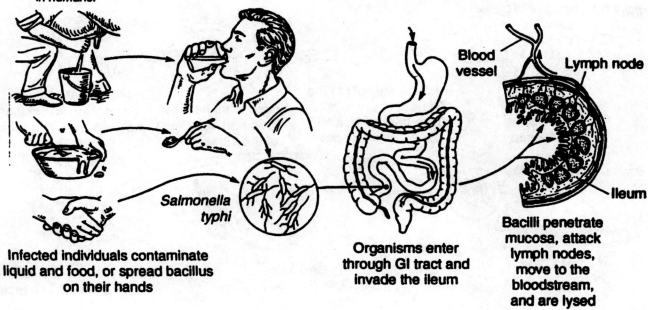

Infected individuals contaminate liquid and food, or spread bacillus on their hands

Salmonella typhi

Organisms enter through GI tract and invade the ileum

Blood vessel

Lymph node

Ileum

Bacilli penetrate mucosa, attack lymph nodes, move to the bloodstream, and are lysed

---

DESCRIPTION: *Salmonella typhi* is a gram-negative, motile, facultatively anaerobic bacillus. It is transmitted through water or milk supplies contaminated by feces of affected people. After contracting the disease, persons may recover but then become chronic carriers. Carriers of the organism, especially food handlers, may be responsible for increased spread of infection. The organisms enter through the GI tract, penetrate the intestinal lining and attack the intestinal lymphoid tissues. From here they enter the lymph vessels and then the bloodstream. In the bloodstream they lyse and release endotoxins which manifest the disease. Surviving bacilli localize in the gallbladder, bone marrow, and spleen. Eventually they return to reinfect the GI tract.

SIGNS AND SYMPTOMS: Fever, abdominal tenderness and distention, bowel disturbances and toxemia are some signs of typhoid fever. Skin eruptions also appear all over the body, and each spot contains viable bacilli. Serious complications of the condition are intestinal hemorrhage and perforation which occur in 25% of the cases and are responsible for the majority of deaths.

LABORATORY DIAGNOSIS: The preferred method of diagnosis is isolation of *S. typhi* from a blood culture, which is positive in most patients during the first two weeks of illness. Urine and stool cultures are positive less frequently, but should be attempted. The Widal test for agglutinating antibodies against the somatic (O) and flagellar (H) antigens of *S. typhi* is widely used for serodiagnosis.

PREVENTION AND TREATMENT: Since non-ill carriers exist, it is important to detect these carriers and to keep them away from food preparation. Prevention can also include maintaining a pure water supply, using only clean, pasteurized milk, and general sanitary control. All items that come in contact with an ill patient should be disinfected. A typhoid vaccine is available and is administered in two doses several weeks apart. It has many side effects, however, so it is advisable only for those who will be exposed to *S. typhi* bacilli. Infection provides permanent immunity in 98% of all cases. Chloramphenicol or ampicillin are the antibiotics of choice.

Typhus Fever (ti'fus) Gk. *typhos*, fever

DEFINITION: Any of a group of acute, infectious diseases caused by related arthropod-borne species of *Rickettsia*. Epidemic typhus is prevalent amid unsanitary conditions and in crowded living conditions.

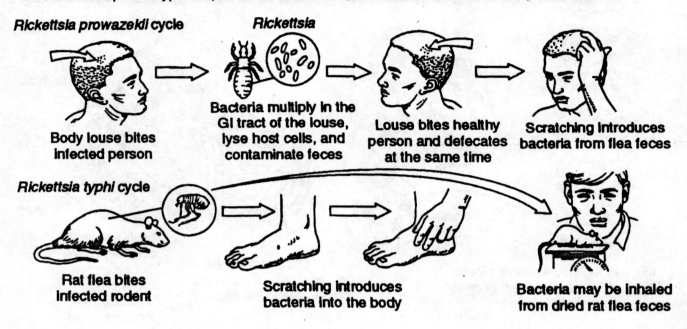

Rickettsia prowazekii cycle

Rickettsia

Body louse bites infected person

Bacteria multiply in the GI tract of the louse, lyse host cells, and contaminate feces

Louse bites healthy person and defecates at the same time

Scratching introduces bacteria from flea feces

Rickettsia typhi cycle

Rat flea bites infected rodent

Scratching introduces bacteria into the body

Bacteria may be inhaled from dried rat flea feces

DESCRIPTION: The typhus fever group includes epidemic typhus, murine typhus, and Brill-Zinsser disease. Epidemic typhus is caused by *Rickettsia prowazekii* and is spread from person to person by the body louse *Pediculus humanus corporis*. The louse bites an ill person and the organisms move to its stomach and invade the intestinal tract lining. They multiply to such an extent that the cells become very swollen and burst, liberating the *Rickettsiae* into the feces of the louse. When the louse bites another person it defecates at the same time. The site of the bite itches and the infectious material is introduced into the skin by scratching. Epidemic typhus is an acute and severe disease with 10–40% mortality. Murine typhus, caused by *R. typhi*, is relatively mild and is transferred to humans by the rat flea. Brill-Zinsser disease is also a mild form of typhus that occurs in persons who have had classic typhus fever many years before. It is caused by *R. prowazekii*.

SIGNS AND SYMPTOMS: Epidemic typhus is characterized by sudden onset, severe headache, pain in the back and limbs and prostration. Sustained high fever is also common as well as bluish spots on the abdomen. The tongue may be covered in a whitish film and in severe, prolonged cases the tongue becomes black and is rolled up at the back of the mouth. Complications include bronchopneumonia and nephritis.

LABORATORY DIAGNOSIS: Diagnosis is made using serodiagnostic tests to detect anti-rickettsial antibodies.

PREVENTION AND TREATMENT: Important prevention techniques include cleanliness, delousing, and insecticides to destroy the vector. Overcrowding should be avoided whenever possible. The disease is most common in areas where living conditions are unfavorable such as army camps and on shipboard. Vaccines are recommended for travelers going to the endemic areas. Broad spectrum antibiotics can be very helpful if given soon enough after infection. Patients with the disease should be isolated, given rest and a liquid diet. Individuals are generally immune after recovery.

Vaginitis (vaj-in-i'tis) L. *vagina*, sheath/ Gk. *itis*, inflammation

DEFINITION: Inflammation of the vagina caused by infection with a variety of microorganisms. It may occur as a result of uncleanliness or sexual transmission from an infected partner.

Sources of infection

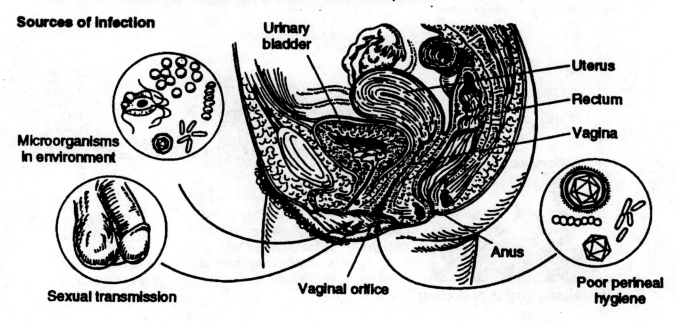

DESCRIPTION: Vaginitis may occur as the result of a variety of infections. Some of the common microorganisms involved include: gonococci, *Chlamydia*, *Candida*, *Gardnerella vaginalis*, staphylococci, streptococci, spirochetes, and viruses. The protozoan flagellate, *Trichomonas vaginalis*, is found in 30–40% of all cases. Herpes simplex viruses are another dangerous cause of inflammation, and the greatest risk involved with herpes concerns the fetus of an infected woman. Some organisms may invade the uterus, or the fetus may contract an infection during delivery. If sepsis develops, then death of the fetus or the baby could result rather quickly due to their undeveloped immune system.

SIGNS AND SYMPTOMS: Some infections may be asymptomatic. When symptoms do occur, however, they include a purulent vaginal discharge which may be malodorous, irritation and itching of the vulva and perineum, and reddened vaginal mucosa. When the cause is *Gardnerella* "*clue cells*" may be present, which are vaginal epithelial cells coated with coccobacilli. There is an increase in the frequency of urination and voiding may be painful. Papilloma virus infections may lead to neoplasm, or cancer of the genital tract.

LABORATORY DIAGNOSIS: Wet mounts in saline and 10% KOH are prepared and examined by direct microscopy. *T. vaginalis* and *C. albicans* can be recognized in fresh specimens, and clue cells may indicate *Gardnerella*. Bacteriologic cultures should be performed to detect *Gardnerella*, *N. gonorrhoeae*, or other pathogens.

PREVENTION AND TREATMENT: Improved perineal hygiene must be learned and practiced. The anus should be cleaned (wiped) from front to back after a bowel movement. Careful partner choice for sexual activity and the use of condoms may further reduce the chance of infection. Treatment includes the use of antimicrobial agents depending on the microorganism involved. Delivery of antibiotics may be orally and/or by suppositories. Dilute vinegar douches are helpful in treating bacterial vaginitis if inflammation is minimal.

Verruca (Wart) (ver-roo'ka) L. *verruca*, wart

DEFINITION: Projections that spring from the skin and are covered with stratified squamous epithelium. They are caused by *papillomaviruses*, many are relatively benign. The cutaneous elevations result from hypertrophy of the papillae and epidermis.

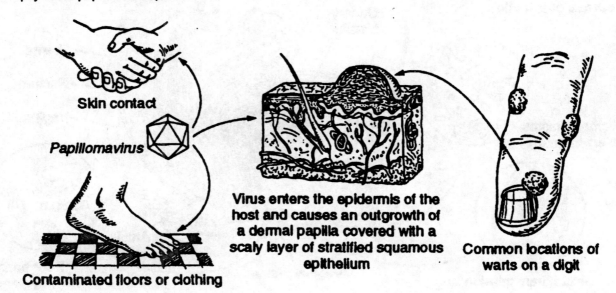

Skin contact

Papillomavirus

Contaminated floors or clothing

Virus enters the epidermis of the host and causes an outgrowth of a dermal papilla covered with a scaly layer of stratified squamous epithelium

Common locations of warts on a digit

DESCRIPTION: Warts are viral tumors derived from the epithelium which are spread by skin contact, contaminated floors and clothing, or coitus (sexual intercourse). A small lesion or abrasion is probably necessary for viral access into the host. The hands and the soles of the feet are common sites for warts. There are a variety of types of warts each caused by a different papilloma virus type. Hand warts (*verucca vulgaris*) are benign growths that increase in size very slowly and usually do not recur after removal. They are well delineated and cause little tissue destruction. Warts on the soles of the feet are called *plantar warts*. *Venereal warts* (*condyloma*) are also seen, particularly on persons who have multiple sexual partners. They occur around the genitalia and anus. Untreated venereal warts may be responsible for some cases of uterine cervical carcinoma.

SIGNS AND SYMPTOMS: A hard, tight concentration of epithelial tissue appears first and slowly grows larger and can project out from the skin. Warts are usually not painful, however plantar warts can become very painful because of the constant pressure applied to them through walking. Warts vary in appearance including some which are red and flat. Certain types of warts are present only in specific family lines, suggesting genetic susceptibility of papilloma virus infection or gene expression.

LABORATORY DIAGNOSIS: To date, human papilloma viruses are not culturable in the laboratory. If desired, wart tissue can be tested with specific DNA probes to determine the presence of virus genomes and to type the causative virus.

PREVENTION AND TREATMENT: Except for venereal warts, verruca are usually self-limiting and may spontaneously and suddenly regress and disappear. This feature has encouraged a vast number of folk medical cures for warts all of which seem to "work" some of the time. Warts can be medically removed by using a sharp spoon curet under local anesthesia. If they are elevated, they may also be clipped off with sharp scissors and treated with a touch of iodine. Freezing warts with liquid nitrogen, treating them with electrocautery, or application of salicylic acid are some other methods of removal. These treatments can be painful but are quite commonly practiced because warts are considered unsightly. Venereal warts should always be medically treated.

Viral Gastroenteritis Gk. *gaster*, stomach; *enteron*, intestine; *itis*, inflamed

DEFINITION: An inflammation of the mucosa of the stomach and intestinal tract due to a viral infection. Although viral gastroenteritis is also called 24-hour flu or intestinal flu, it is not caused by the *H. influenzae* bacteria, nor influenza virus.

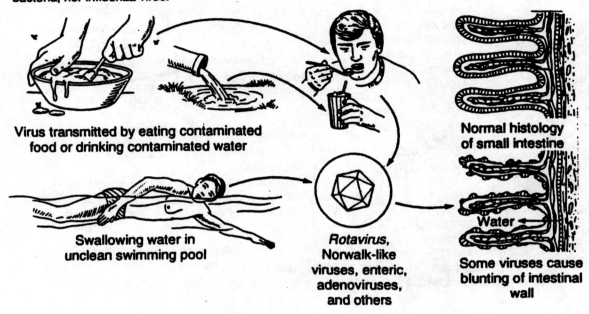

Virus transmitted by eating contaminated food or drinking contaminated water

Swallowing water in unclean swimming pool

Rotavirus, Norwalk-like viruses, enteric, adenoviruses, and others

Normal histology of small intestine

Water

Some viruses cause blunting of intestinal wall

DESCRIPTION: Viral gastroenteritis is transmitted through the fecal-oral route. Thus if proper sanitation and handwashing practices are not followed, contaminated foods handled or processed by a person having the disease can become sources of infection. Viral gastroenteritis may also be contracted from consumption of contaminated drinking water and swallowing water in unclean swimming pools. The condition is more common during winter months. *Rotavirus*, a genus in the family *Reoviridae*, causes infantile gastroenteritis which is common in developing countries and a major cause of infant deaths. A variety of *parvoviruses* may cause gastroenteritis in adults. Also, the *Norwalk group* of viruses, classified tentatively as *Caliciviruses*, are proven etiologic agents of gastroenteritis. In addition, many kinds of enteric adenoviruses, small round viruses, astroviruses, and icosahedral viruses have been seen by electron microscopy in stool filtrates from infected people. The Norwalk group of viruses cause blunting of the intestinal villi and inflammatory changes which reduce the activity of digestive enzymes. The mechanism of the viral action is unknown.

SIGNS AND SYMPTOMS: Viral gastroenteritis has an acute onset which includes fever, loss of appetite, abdominal pain, vomiting, and diarrhea. Illness usually lasts only 12–24 hours. A child under two years of age may have prolonged symptoms and severe dehydration.

LABORATORY DIAGNOSIS: Rotavirus infections are diagnosed by direct antigen detection EIA or latex agglutination tests. Enteric adenovirus infections are detected by EIA antigen determination tests, and other viruses are detected by immune electron microscopy or simple electron microscopy.

PREVENTION AND TREATMENT: Basic sanitary practices can limit the spread of the disease. Immune mothers can confer a temporary immunity to their babies through breast milk. Recovery from infant gastroenteritis may confer immunity. There is only a short-term, type specific immunity for adults. No vaccine or specific treatment is available for any type of viral gastroenteritis.

Yellow Fever

DEFINITION: A hemorrhagic fever in which jaundice, or a yellow discoloration of the skin, is characteristic; caused by a mosquito-borne *flavivirus* (L. *flavus*, yellow).

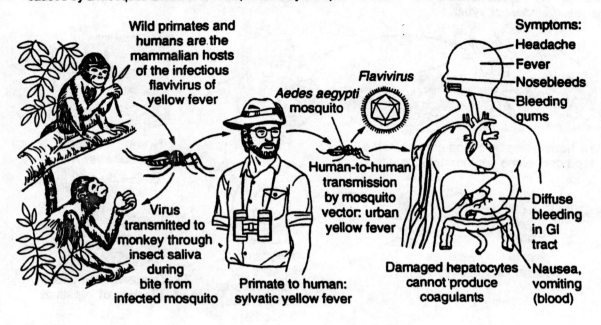

Wild primates and humans are the mammalian hosts of the infectious flavivirus of yellow fever

Flavivirus

Aedes aegypti mosquito

Virus transmitted to monkey through insect saliva during bite from infected mosquito

Primate to human: sylvatic yellow fever

Human-to-human transmission by mosquito vector: urban yellow fever

Damaged hepatocytes cannot produce coagulants

Symptoms:
- Headache
- Fever
- Nosebleeds
- Bleeding gums
- Diffuse bleeding in GI tract
- Nausea, vomiting (blood)

DESCRIPTION: The yellow fever virus is spherical and 40–50 nm in diameter. Its single-stranded RNA genome is contained in the icosahedral nucleocapsid. The virus generally infects monkeys in the tropical forests of Central Africa and Central and South America, and human infection is primarily confined to people in contact with these forest areas. A variety of mosquito species may transmit the disease to humans, but *Aedes aegypti* is the principal vector in person-to-person transmission. After a mosquito feeds on the blood of an infected primate, infectious viral particles develop in its salivary glands in 8 to 12 days, and the mosquito remains infectious throughout the rest of its 6 to 8 week lifetime. When an infected mosquito bites a human, the virus enters the bloodstream directly, and after a 3 to 7 day incubation period, infects tissues throughout the body. In particular, the liver cells are damaged to the point that they cannot synthesize coagulation proteins. This accounts for the diverse bleeding which categorizes yellow fever among "hemorrhagic" fevers.

SIGNS AND SYMPTOMS: The symptoms of yellow fever are distinct over an eight day period.

Days 1–3	Sudden fever, nausea, vomiting, headache, backache, some jaundice
Days 3–4	Period of remission, varying from a number of hours to two days
Days 5–8	Symptoms reappear with greater severity, pronounced jaundice, patient exhibits "black vomit" (partially digested blood from severe stomach hemorrhage), nosebleeds and bleeding gums

In severe cases, the patient will experience renal failure, followed by coma and death six to eight days after onset. Although the majority of yellow fever cases are mild, the mortality rate from the disease is about 20%.

LABORATORY DIAGNOSIS: Diagnosis is made by isolation of yellow fever virus from the blood or detection of a rising antibody titer.

PREVENTION AND TREATMENT: Vaccination and the use of protective clothing and insect repellents are effective in prevention. Mosquitoes are eradicated using insecticides. No specific treatment for yellow fever exists, but the antiviral drug ribavirin may be effective. Blood transfusions may help to control bleeding.

Flatworms

DEFINITION: Freshwater and parasitic soft-bodied, flattened animals within the phylum *Platyhelminthes* (about 15,000 species); includes planaria, flukes, and tapeworms.

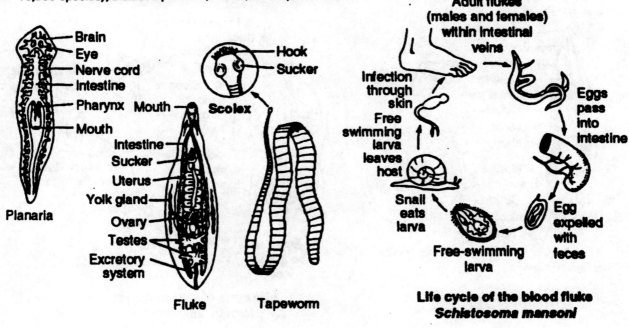

Life cycle of the blood fluke *Schistosoma mansoni*

DESCRIPTION: Flatworms are elongated, flattened, and are *bilaterally symmetrical*. The flatworm body is composed of three tissue layers (ectoderm, mesoderm, and endoderm), and has a distinct head with a simple brain consisting of two masses of nervous tissue called *ganglia*. *Nerve cords* from the ganglia extend the length of the body. Excretory organs, called *protonephridia*, consist of *flame cells* in the body tissues and branched *tubules* that extend through the body and exit through *pores* at the body surface. When present, the mouth opens into the *gastrovascular cavity*. The reproductive organs are well developed.

Representative kinds	Characteristics
Class Turbellaria: planarians	Mostly free-living, carnivorous, aquatic forms; body covered by ciliated epidermis
Class Trematoda: flukes (e.g., schistosomes)	Parasitic with wide range of invertebrate and vertebrate hosts; suckers for attachment to host
Class Cestoda: tapeworms	Parasitic on many vertebrate hosts; complex life cycle with intermediate hosts; suckers or hooks on scolex for attachment to host; eggs produced and shed within proglottids

APPLICATION: Because the human is a host animal for many flatworms, these parasitic animals are of major health concern in tropical countries where they cause high numbers of deaths, especially in children. Parasitic flatworms absorb significant quantities of nutrients, secrete toxic wastes, and generally interfere with the host's normal physiological processes.

Roundworms

DEFINITION: A wide variety of small, elongated animals within the phylum *Nematoda* (about 80,000 species); includes many free-living forms in water and soil, and parasitic forms such as hookworms, pinworms, *Ascaris*, and *Trichinella*.

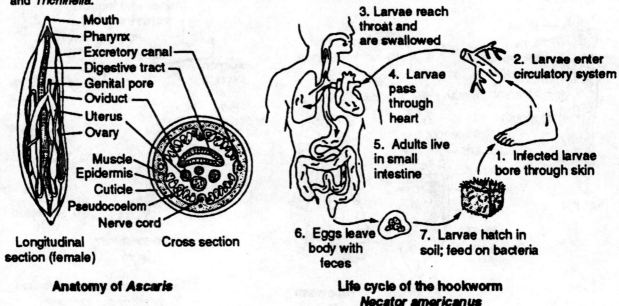

Anatomy of *Ascaris*

Longitudinal section (female)

Cross section

- Mouth
- Pharynx
- Excretory canal
- Digestive tract
- Genital pore
- Oviduct
- Uterus
- Ovary
- Muscle
- Epidermis
- Cuticle
- Pseudocoelom
- Nerve cord

Life cycle of the hookworm *Necator americanus*

3. Larvae reach throat and are swallowed
4. Larvae pass through heart
5. Adults live in small intestine
2. Larvae enter circulatory system
1. Infected larvae bore through skin
6. Eggs leave body with feces
7. Larvae hatch in soil; feed on bacteria

DESCRIPTION: Mostly microscopic, nematodes are bilaterally symmetrical, cylindrical, unsegmented worms. The body of a nematode is enclosed in a tough *cuticle* that is shed periodically as the animal grows. Contraction of the longitudinal skeletal muscles attached to the cuticle causes a shiplike body movement. Nematodes lack smooth muscle and have an incomplete mesodermal layer. The body cavity is called a *pseudocoelom* because it is not totally lined with mesoderm. The tubular digestive tract extends the length of the body from the *mouth* to the *anus*. The sexes are usually separate, and the female is larger than the male.

APPLICATION: The estimated thousands of nematodes in a spadeful of soil are primary consumers of organic materials. They are also extremely important in marine and freshwater food chains. Other nematodes are parasites of plants and animals. Among the human nematode parasites are the hookworms, the intestinal roundworm *Ascaris*, pinworms, trichina worms (*Trichinella*), and filarial worms.

Elephantiasis caused by filarial worms blocking the lymphatic drainage

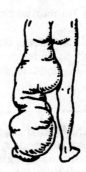